I Create My Day

*Simple ways to create
a beautiful and nourishing life*

Veronika Sophia Robinson

Starflower Press

I Create My Day: *Simple ways to create a beautiful and nourishing life*
© Written by Veronika Sophia Robinson
© Cover illustration by Tracy Jane Roper
ISBN 978-0-9931586-2-9
Published by Starflower Press ~ February 2016
www.starflowerpress.com
British Library Cataloguing in Publication Data. A catalogue record for this book is available from the British Library.

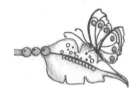

Author's Note

It always amuses me how books come into being. The main character in my novel, *Sisters of the Silver Moon*, is Azaria Linden. For the most part, she lives a charmed life. When one of my readers said to me that she wanted a life like that, and 'could I write a book telling her how to do it?', I laughed. Although Azaria is fictional, the way she lives her life can be achieved. This book sets out to give you a template. You, however, have to do the daily work.

Creating your day is empowering, rewarding and lifechanging. Are you up for it? Come on, then! I invite you to start getting out of bed on the right side every day.

Thank you!

Thank you to Tracy for creating the lovely cover art. It is a joy collaborating with you, and I look forward to many more joint projects.

Mum, thank you for being such an inspirational light in my childhood, and for teaching me the fundamental truth: *I am a creator*.

Paul, for being part of my every day, and bringing such pleasure and contentment to my life. Your creative expression is always a joy to witness.

Denise Ridgway, for asking me to write this book! I hope it doesn't disappoint.

Fleur Parker, for your review of *Sisters of the Silver Moon* on Amazon. When you wrote the words "Veronika creates my day", a light switched on inside. Thank you.

My daughters, Beth and Eliza, for being such awesome creations to come out of my body. Mostly, though, for being such inspiring examples of the beauty of creativity.

Beth, may your love of creating and composing music be a guiding force throughout your whole life. Thank you so much for the pleasure you have brought me.

Eliza, I trust that the powerful words you write continue to grow and blossom and find the perfect readers. May you both always have the applause of a grateful audience.

To you, the reader, for attracting this book into your life. Be inspired. Go create!

For my first grandchild.

May you discover that to create is the greatest joy of all.

I wish you an amazing and beautiful life.
Welcome to our family.

Love, Oma xxx

CONTENTS

Morning has broken
Like the first morning.
Blackbird has spoken
Like the first bird
Praise for the singing, praise for the morning…

*You have the power
to create your day.*

Good Morning

"When you arise in the morning,
think of what a precious privilege it is to be alive;
to breathe, to think, to enjoy, to love."
~ Marcus Aurelius

Good morning! What a beautiful new day. The birds are singing, the Sun is rising over the hills outside my bedroom, and the fields are covered in dew. I feel such joy in my heart. It's great to be alive!

Maybe you don't feel that way. Perhaps you start each day with dread, and your first thought is: Crap, another day.

Are you someone who suffers low-grade anxiety even if nothing bad is happening in your life?

What if it didn't have to be this way? Have you ever considered that life doesn't have to be a constant struggle? That, perhaps, we're here on this Earth to live and grow with joy? I hope you'll stay with me as I share how you can create a life worth living and loving.

The human brain is incredibly powerful. Most people input negative information, dozens of times a day, and then wonder why they have unsatisfying lives. Thinking of your brain as a computer can give you the shift you need to instigate huge life changes.

The more you enter data that expresses the life you want to live, the quicker everything will change. Many of us have been indoctrinated to live according to what our parents, teachers, friends, religion or culture would have us believe. When we start making choices that suit our inner calling, our life can change in seemingly miraculous ways.

Every day is sacred. You and I will never walk through this day again. Let's celebrate this wonderful earthly existence by creating more beauty, more bounty and more love. Who wouldn't want that?

Before I open my eyes in the morning, I give thanks. I say "I am so grateful for this beautiful life". The feeling of gratitude overwhelms me.

I thank my body. I thank my comfy bed and pillow. I thank the new day. I thank the birds for their enchanting songs. Isn't it funny how they never wake up in a bad mood and decide not to sing?

I express gratitude that my husband is alive and well beside me. I am thankful that my daughters are healthy. I am appreciative that I do work that I love.

After I give thanks, I think through my day, such as what plans I have, and how I want things to proceed. I literally create my day before I have even got out of bed. *I expect the best.* I am open to good and wonderful things coming into my life. I am suggestible to kindness, laughter, peace, friendship, prosperity and good health.

If we start our day with the heartfelt expectation that we wish to be living the highest version of ourselves,

Your heart literally has the power to give your brain new commands.

then our intention has no choice but to manifest.

Before we 'do' our day, it helps to think, visualise and create the day in our mind and heart.

The brain and heart have direct nerve connections. In fact, there are many more that go from the heart to the brain than from the brain to the heart. We take from this that it's important to 'feel' our way into any changes we want to make. Your heart literally has the power to give your brain new commands. Think about that for a moment, and how incredibly empowering that is for anyone wanting to live intentionally. The heart has an electromagnetic field that reaches out to the farthest reaches of the Universe. This means we can literally feed off that cosmic energy and manifest miracles in our lives.

If you've not lived with deliberate intention like this before, remember this: the body is based on chemical reactions. *You have the power to shift these.* You have the power to create your day. You're not a victim of Fate unless you choose to be.

You do, however, have to be consistent with any new practice until it becomes a habit. As you put these ideas into play, you'll notice the Universe acknowledging you with many acts of seeming coincidence. Don't dismiss them. Rejoice in each declaration.

If there's one thing I truly believe, it is this: *we are here on Earth to discover our creativity, and to live with pleasure.* That is all.

This book is an invitation to you to live an intentional life. I hope you will accept.

Heart Questions

How do you feel when waking up in the morning?
Do you look forward to each new day?
Do you love Mondays, or dread them?
Do you feel like it is possible to change your life for the better?
Do you feel empowered on your journey through life, or like a victim of circumstance?
What steps can you take to create a life where you bounce out of bed in the morning with gratitude and enthusiasm?

Until further notice,
celebrate everything!

*I choose to manifest
consciously and with integrity.*

The First Hour

The first hour of the day is your power point. The morning is governed by Spring, and ruled by Aries, the zodiac sign of action. This first hour or so belongs to your vision of life, and your deepest dreams. Keep it sacrosanct.

Humans are creatures of habit, for better or worse. We have the ability to completely transform our lives by committing to a new plan of action. When we make changes which serve to nourish us, short and long term, then such habits provide the sustenance which feeds body and soul.

When my daughter Eliza was a toddler, she started every morning by asking me "what are we doing that's fun today?" Ha! No pressure. She proved to be an incredible teacher, and taught me that it was an important question for each of us.

Consider beginning the day with questions such as:

What can I do to laugh today?
What fun can I manifest today?
What kindnesses can I bring to someone's day?
Where can I express gratitude today?
How can I be a more loving person today?

The morning is such a powerful time because we are fresh from sleep: that place where we're connected to our Higher Self. I highly recommend using this narrow window of time to embed new ways of thinking and being. The connection between this world and the Source from Whence We Came, in the first hour of the day, is extraordinarily strong. Ironically, it's the time that the vast majority of people in our culture cling to caffeine, highly processed breakfast cereals, and watch the news. These are particularly damaging to us during this sensitive psychic time frame.

The news teaches us that the world is a dangerous and unfriendly place. What if you replaced that source of information with inspirational reading, poetry, walking barefoot on Mother Earth, meditation, yoga, prayer, affirmations, a cup of herbal tea, lovemaking, or an early-morning swim? How might your life feel then?

Stress is created by resistance, so it's important to go with the flow if you expect to live a happy and charmed life. In each circumstance of your day, take a moment to ask 'what am I learning from this?' 'Am I responding as the highest version of myself?'

If someone is going through a tough time, avoid shaming them, or yourself, by asking "why did you create that?" It's not helpful! If someone has been diagnosed with an illness, for example, they need your support not your judgement.

We're all learning, and we're all making our way in the world. In short, we are all apprentices with the potential to become masters of intentional living.

Creating your day isn't just about what you do, but about what you don't do. It's a delicious dance between action and inaction, between movement and stillness.

In the moments of quiet, we go inwards and connect

with our place in the world. We make time to honour ourselves and those around us. Simple daily habits and rituals bring our attention to the parts of life we wish to amplify. Small rituals allow us to establish routines and rhythms which nurture us, our home, and the other spaces around us. They become foundations for the building of our day, and our lives.

The time you devote to your morning rhythm is the template of your day. Simple actions can create calm, love, balance, groundedness, and poise. They can also eliminate chaos. Look, too, to your bedtime, and your rituals around that. One part of the day sets the tone for the hours ahead, and the other offers us a chance to close the current day and prepare for the next. Sunrise. Sunset. Open. Close. Your rituals need to be personal to you, and ideas and practices that you're comfortable with, or can grow to find comforting.

I learnt the hard, and health-damaging, way that stress is a choice. Joy and calm are choices, too. Take your pick. We may not be able to control certain situations, such as a death or weather conditions, but we *always*, in any given circumstance, have a choice about how to respond. This is where our power lies.

Your daily rhythm will ideally be filled with love, and reverence, be empowering, and nourish you deeply. By creating habits that support you in this way, you'll see your life transform.

This day is our greatest gift. How, then, shall we write upon it? I love the idea of a blank slate, and creating my dreams and hopes upon it. How about you? Does it fill you with joy and excitement?

Each day, like sheaves of an accordion, leads right up to the next one which follows, and backs into the one behind. How we value the quality of our life rests upon

The time you devote to your morning rhythm is the template of your day.

how we spend each day. Contrary to popular belief, a good life isn't marked just by major events such as buying a home, getting a pay rise or getting married. A wonderful, soul-filled life is one whereby every waking day is a pleasure. The ordinary day becomes extraordinary.

Life is not to be survived, but something whereby we thrive. How we do that is based not on what life throws our way, but how we create and how we respond.

If today was a template of your lifetime, how would you spend it?

This book hopes to have you asking this question often enough that you begin each day knowing that you're a creator.

Scattered like rose-petal confetti throughout this book are tips, ideas, rituals, remedies, affirmations and personal stories for creating a life you can love. I hope they inspire you.

By catching the worm and being up with the early bird, you end up making significant changes in your life. That's not to say you should never sleep in, or enjoy a cosy rendezvous with your lover between the sheets, but making a practice of greeting the day with the Sun can give you a new perspective. I never thought of myself as an early-morning person until I became one for practical reasons. For years I was a home-educating mother of two while editing an international natural-parenting magazine, and writing books; and I needed to establish time that was 'just mine'. I find mornings peaceful and quiet, and I am at my most productive then.

I know that nourishing yourself through body-friendly foods and liquids will fuel your day in many ways.

The gym is not my natural habitat. I'd much rather enjoy a solitary walk through the woods. However, by going to the leisure centre most days, and doing swimming, aquafit, workouts in the gym, or a dynamic-control-and-stretch class, I have become one of those people which studies suggest is calmer, able to cope better with life, and is happier.

Go on, go for a twenty minute walk right now and see how much better you feel afterwards. I'm not kidding. Put the book down.

Did you do it? Where did you go? The beach? An Irish bog? Wildflower meadow? City park? Canal path? Snow-covered fallow field? A deep dark forest? What did you see? What experiences did you have? How did you feel? Are you invigorated?

At the heart of living a life you love is actually making sure you spend time doing activities that bring you pleasure and make you feel energised.

Most of us live in a state of socially acceptable exhaustion, and are fuelled by caffeine, TV, social media, and junk foods. Our bodies were not designed for modern living. Besides nutritious fuel, we need rest. It's okay to put your feet up. It's okay to have a siesta. And, it's perfectly okay to go to bed early. The world won't stop just because you're looking after yourself.

Don't be shamed into living a life of sleep deprivation. It's not worth it.

Be mindful, not just of your day, but of those people you interact with, whether they're companions or strangers. Make eye contact. Walk with your head held high and a smile on your face. Put your mobile phone down or away. Be present.

Your soul needs nurturing. This isn't something you can only do in a church or a temple, but an everyday practice based on faith, gratitude, beauty and love.

My wish is that as you work your way through this book, you will create a home and a life to nourish you, as well as faith, optimism, simplicity and patience. I trust that you will learn to cherish the unhurried life.

I firmly believe, and know from my own experience, that by taking time each day to deliberately and consciously create your day, you will grow spiritually and feel connected to the Universe, flourish in all areas of your life, create robust health, and develop an inner strength that will take you through trying times. May your inner growth be reflected in the life you live, and the life you love. Slow living enables us to relish, enjoy, savour and cherish this precious life.

*"Success in life is founded upon attention
to the small things rather than to the large things."*
~ Booker T. Washington

> **TIP:** *Before going to sleep, do a quick declutter so that your home feels fresh when you wake up in the morning.*

What are you going to do today to make your day beautiful, love filled, amazing and joyous?
1
2
3
4
5

What are you grateful for today?
1
2
3
4
5

Choose five positive thoughts about yourself for today.
I am…
I am…
I am…
I am…
I am…

To create your day, develop habits that can/will lead to creating the life you want. Many goals simply don't get achieved overnight. They take dedication, perseverance, responsibility and patience. But remember this: actions always speak louder than words.

If today were a template of your lifetime, how would you spend it?

Creating your day is one of the greatest spiritual decisions you can make. As you deliberately set the tone and intention of your day, coincidences and serendipity will knock at your door. Welcome them in!

Recognise that you have unlimited potential to create the life and dreams of your heart.

Start each day with the words: *I create my day.* Say them out loud, or say them in your mind.

Let's be clear: even if you are creating your day, and are positive and upbeat, incidences may come along that were not part of your conscious plan. Regardless of the reason they have turned up in your life, what you do have is the ability to create your *reaction* to any and all situations, no matter how dramatic or tragic or even mundane. The choice in how we perceive a situation is determined within our inner realm. Your internal landscape need not be tarnished, temporarily or permanently, by an outer event.

Always Look on the Bright Side

Studies show that optimistic people create good luck for themselves. Conversely, pessimists don't believe they're lucky, and have a hard time bringing joy into their lives. It is a person's optimism—their faith in life and the future—which makes them resilient to life's knocks. They are living proof that you literally create your own luck.

Intuition

Trust that inner voice. The more you listen and act on that still voice within, the more it will speak to you.

Set Goals and Write Lists

I do believe one of the key strategies for creating the life of your dreams is to write down your goals. Working towards dreams, big and small, is more likely to happen when we put them into black and white.

When you say or write the words *I create my day*, you are sending a strong message to the Universe. You are speaking truth. By engaging in this act, you must be open to watching your life manifest according to your desires. Two of the most important words we can speak are *I am*. Choose carefully the words you speak after them, such as I am tired. I am angry. I am broke.

Always make the words you use after *I am* positive and empowering.

One of the things I disagree with is the use of the affirmation *I am an alcoholic* in Alcoholics Anonymous. I do understand the idea of people taking responsibility for their actions, but when a person constantly says out loud *I am an alcoholic,* they are affirming their disease over and over again. Perhaps someone has been an alcoholic, but surely in the interests of healing there is a better way to use language?

I am sober. How different does that sound? It is liberating, empowering, positive. *I am healed. I am healthy. I am balanced.* Or, as a work in progress, *I am recovering.* These carry such a different vibration.

I hope, at some point, AA finds a new way to support its members into remembering and activating their wholeness. This isn't about denial, but renewal, growth, faith and trust.

When you start your day, be sure to include a nourishing breakfast as part of your morning ritual. If you don't feel hungry first thing in the morning, it's highly possible that your liver is not functioning as well as it could. It is a sign of good health to wake up feeling hungry.

Be aware that when taking in food and beverages, this isn't the time to be imbibing the latest murder or Wall Street catastrophe. Eat your food in silence or pleasurable companionship. Your digestive system will thank you for it.

Beginning your day by expecting the best sends a message out to the Universe. Consciously express kindness and tolerance to everyone you come in contact with, whether it's by phone, on the road, or face to face. Engage your smile muscles as if your life depends on them.

I grew up with a beautiful wall poster in the kitchen of our childhood home:

A smile costs nothing, but gives much.
It enriches those who receive,
without making poorer those who give.
It takes but a moment,
but the memory of it sometimes lasts forever.

Give your smiles freely. Feed yourself, and other people, with love and affection. Nourish your mind, body and soul with beauty, respect and integrity. Engage in pleasurable activities which honour body and soul.

A key factor to consciously creating each day is that of living in the present moment. By being 100% focused on where you are, who you're with, and what you're doing, you open yourself up to living with grace. We

*Creating your day
is one of the greatest
spiritual decisions
you can make.*

may not be able to see the future, but we sure can create it.

Those who walk this journey learn that less is more, and that the secret ingredient to a love-filled, soul-felt life is often about doing less in the external world and more inner work.

What happens when we start refining our dreams and goals is that we come to narrow down our wishes into key areas. With laser-like focus, we manifest our dreams into reality. On that foundation, we start to build our life.

For example, your goals might be:

Create a beautiful home
Excellent health and well-being
Vibrant marriage
Happy parenting
World travel

You would then divide these areas up into doable steps. And each day, you would focus on how to create them the way you feel them in your heart.

For example, perhaps you can find ways to enliven your marriage, such as getting rid of the TV or only watching it two nights a week? What about...

Cooking a meal together?
Going for a walk at sunset each night?
Talking?
Listening. Really listening?
Back or foot massages? (that don't lead to sex)
Enrolling in a night class together?

As you open to the idea of creating a loving and vibrant marriage, new ways of communing and communicating will manifest for you.

Where do you even begin to become a conscious creator? When you wake up (and you can do this before you even open your eyes), give thanks. Express gratitude for anything and everything you can think of, and allow your whole body to move into an expansive and appreciate state. *I am grateful for my health. I am grateful for my family. I am grateful for my beautiful home.*

Raise your vibration by smiling. Try the heart smile. Imagine your heart is literally smiling and spreading right across your chest with joy. Allow a smile across your face. This is a great way to reduce stress, and allows you to manifest easily because your vibration is high.

Before you get out of bed, allow yourself to stretch. This is a simple thing to do that will gently help your body to wake up and come into alignment.

After giving thanks, smiling and stretching, say or think: *I create my day.* Go through your plans for the day and visualise them in the best possible way. If you have no set plans, visualise yourself feeling happy, relaxed, laughing, peaceful.

Heart Questions

What is your morning ritual?
In what ways does it support you (or hold you back from) in living a joyous day?
What steps can you take to bring more consciousness to the first hour of your day?
What daily practices make you smile when you think of incorporating them?
What are you grateful for?
How will/did you spend your day?
How would you have liked to have spent it?

A mini-lesson from William the cat

"Ask and ye shall receive."

William is a master student of manifestation. He knows that he only has to ask and I will deliver him goodies and snacks. If I am too busy making a meal, for example, to listen to his miaows, he'll ask in a new way by tripping me up. He's clear about what he wants, and he'll persist. We can all learn from William.

Conscious Creation

When I worked at a school of metaphysics more than two decades ago, one of the foundation teachings was about conscious creation. You may know it as the Christmas story. Mary meets Joseph, and they have the baby Jesus. Metaphysically, this story is about the feminine, Mary, (*feelings*) joining with the masculine, Joseph, (*thoughts*) and producing (*creating*) the baby Jesus (Christ consciousness). You don't need to be religious or even believe in the Bible to understand the relevance of this story in your own life. Whenever we wish to manifest (create) something in our life, we need to marry our *feelings* with our *thoughts*. When they match, then this *desire* (which means 'of the Father') will bring forth our creation. Whether you choose to consciously create your day through visualisation or written/ spoken affirmations, your feelings and thoughts must be aligned for manifestation to occur.

Heart Questions
Am I a conscious creator?
In what ways do I consciously create my day?
In what ways do I sabotage my chances of having a happy, beautiful and productive day? How does that benefit me?

"An intention is a quality of consciousness that you bring to an action."
~ From *The Seat Of The Soul* by Gary Zukav

My Mother's Morning Ritual

One of the things I've often heard over the years since becoming a mentor for mothers is that they don't have time to even pee, let alone do anything nourishing for themselves.

I know, from experience, that whatever we want more of in life, we have to give. Want more time? *Give* more time. Want more love? *Give* more love. Want more money? *Give* more money.

As a child, I had a great role model in my mother. She raised eight of us, virtually single-handedly as my father worked overseas for months at a time. She was, quite literally, on her own when it came to raising us.

Mum would wake about two or so hours before us children, and in that sacred time before sunrise, she would meditate, and do her yoga asanas outside on the dewy grass. Around sunrise, the power time of the day, she was creating sacred space and time for herself. By the time us children tumbled out of bed, she was in the kitchen squeezing us all fresh orange juice, with classical music playing in the background. My mother was dedicated and disciplined enough to honour the time she needed for herself to be able to function as a woman and a mother, especially at 'rush hour' before we headed off to school.

During the day, she managed a 700-acre horse stud, kept our home immaculate, and grew a flourishing and beautiful four-acre garden. At the risk of making her sound like superwoman (okay, she is!), she created all our wholefood vegetarian meals from scratch. I don't think I ate a takeaway meal till I was about sixteen. We didn't have a nanny or a gardener or a cook. My mother did everything (with the help of us children doing some chores, too).

One of the key distractions and time wasters that my mother didn't have in her life was modern technology as we know it: Internet and mobile phones. Her life wasn't frittered away looking at a screen, but instead, spent living and celebrating each glorious day.

By engaging with life, she managed to pursue her interests of psychological astrology and gardening-by-the-Moon with a passion and deep sense of purpose. She is a profoundly creative woman, and we were blessed to witness her life force manifest before our eyes: cooking, gardening, dressmaking, home-making, woodwork, art and music.

From my mother, I learnt the art of creating sacred ceremonies in everyday living, with reverence for each mouthful of food I ate, and every star I wished upon. At her side, I learnt to affirm: *health, strength and vitality*, as I sipped my freshly made orange juice each morning.

In this life, I have truly experienced the world through my senses. I've felt the ecstasy of walking in a forest after the rain, and breathing in the scent of eucalyptus leaves. The tender touch of a lover has awakened my skin. As I lick sun-ripened mango juice off my fingers, or breathe in the scent of my children's hair when we hug, I love life. By invoking my senses, I have learnt to truly live. I know, with certainty, that we are on this planet to seek out and experience pleasure. It is a fundamental biological need. We do this by engaging our senses, including our sixth sense.

In the quest to create our day, aren't we really asking that we become more alive? Aren't we, quite simply, asking to feel more of life?

I share about my mother here, because it's so easy to think we don't have time to 'consciously create our day'. And yet, how odd, that we have time to unconsciously create our day by worrying, complaining, being fearful, gossiping, jealousy, and spending hours looking at other people's lives on Facebook and Twitter, watching television, and reading blogs. What if that time was invested in your inner life? How differently might you feel about yourself, your family, and your life's purpose?

Heart Questions

How did my mother and father start their day?
What family rituals did we have around the first hour of the day?
Did we have special rituals around food or holidays?
Have I carried on those rituals/habits in my own life?
Do my patterns serve me?

*Complaining
is the opposite
of gratitude.*

Raise Your Vibration

All great teachers throughout time have taught this fundamental truth: *our outer world reflects our inner world.* To manifest more joy, love, laughter, and all the other pleasurable goodies of this amazing life, it is essential to raise our vibration. We then magnetise similar vibrations to what we're emitting.

Use these ideas to help raise your vibration:
[] Say thank you or write a thank-you note.
[] Absorb the beauty around you (your lover's eyes, a child's smile, moonlight, wildflowers, a stream flowing through a mossy woodland, Autumnal sunlight on golden leaves). Remember, beauty can be found anywhere!
[] Activate abundance within you by doing something kind for someone else.
[] Listen to music you love.
[] Dance (like no one is watching).
[] Go for a run.
[] Walk in the woods or anywhere in Nature that feels good to you.
[] Meditate
[] Pray (as in gratitude, not a plea).
[] Play with a pet.

[] Smell flowers.

[] Walk barefoot on the grass.

[] Take time to laugh with a friend.

[] Read something inspirational like *Women Who Run with the Wolves* or anything by Kahlil Gibran.

[] Listen to chants by monks or nuns.

[] Yoga or Pilates.

[] Hug someone for at least a minute, and let the 'love hormone' oxytocin pulse through your veins. No humans about to hug? Try a pet. No pet? Find a tree. No tree? Hug yourself!

[] Collect gifts from Nature, such as berries, shells, cones and leaves, and create a little altar in your home

[] Meet a friend for a cuppa. Avoid gossiping.

[] Blow bubbles. Allow them to land on your nose!

[] Drink a couple of glasses of pure water (this is a fast way to raise your vibe!).

[] Eat living foods (fresh fruits, vegetables, nuts and seeds).

[] Exercise. There are so many to choose from. Find something you enjoy. My favourite is swimming.

[] Sometimes the thing we need most is a nap. Don't apologise for it. My sister, Heidi, has enjoyed afternoon naps for years and years, and swears by it. (Mind you, she's Australian, and swears a lot!)

[] Create your own aromatherapy spa, and enliven your senses with pure essential oils.

[] As a child, I was always climbing trees. Don't undervalue how much fun it is to see the world from a different perspective.

[] Who says adults can't have fun at the playground and play on the swings? Go on! How high can you swing?

[] "Stop daydreaming, Veronika!" my school teachers would yell at me. How wrong they were.

Daydreaming is essential for happiness and creating your own reality. It allows us to live in bliss time, and to rejuvenate. You have my permission to daydream.

[] Live anywhere near the beach? Make a fabulous sandcastle and spend some time really playing.

[] Spray magnesium on your skin each day. This stuff is like a master class in Zen for your cells, and is the ultimate relaxant. Transdermal (through the skin) magnesium is the best way to absorb this essential mineral.

[] Step away from all forms of technology (electromagnetic radiation) and get back into the natural field.

[] Declutter (works every time!)

[] Practise forgiveness (of self and others).

[] Healing modalities: reflexology, floatation tank, massage, craniosacral therapy, shiatsu, for example.

[] Lovemaking (if you're single, read Sex for One: the joy of self-loving).

[] Fly a kite.

[] Plant some flower or vegetable seeds.

[] Bake a cake.

[] Bathe in moonlight.

[] Stop complaining, even about the weather.

[] Your vibe attracts your tribe! Choose company wisely (it is said we become like the five people we hang out with the most).

[] Watch a comedy. There's nothing like laughing out loud to shift your vibe up several notches.

[] I loved to skip as a child. It's a very different energy to running. Try skipping. It's fun.

[] Thump your thymus (see page 189)

After he was expelled from school for rebelling against rote learning, Einstein began his theory of relativity while daydreaming about riding, or running beside a sunbeam to the edge of the Universe.

What can I do to raise my vibration?

1.
2.
3.
4.
5.
6.
7.
8.
9.
10.

Heart Questions

Do I actively and consciously choose pleasure and delight in my life?
What are my favourite scents?
What is my favourite food?
What is my favourite music?
What sounds bring me the most pleasure?
In what ways do I regularly nourish myself?

Flower Essences

I'm a firm believer in the potency of flower essences as a healing modality. These gifts from the earth allow us to marry their energy with those of the sky (astrology), and bring great healing.

Oftentimes, when we embark on a path of healing we have subconscious issues which prevent or slow it down. Flower essences restore balance on the etheric and emotional levels. Major blocks shift, and life can change in miraculous ways when remedies are taken. For others, the shift may be subtle.

Edward Bach described the flower remedies: "They cure, not by attacking disease, but by flooding our bodies with the beautiful vibrations of our Higher Nature, in the presence of which disease melts as snow in the sunshine".

Self-medicating with flower essences provides us with an excellent self-help resource. They are deeply empowering, and don't require a practitioner. I recommend them as a way to help us listen to the wise voice within, and to live more in the flow of life.

Two men looked out
from prison bars.
One saw mud
and one saw stars.

The Creator

We are all creators, it's just that some of us do so deliberately by *setting our intentions,* and then focusing on them. Other people also create their lives, but don't understand how powerful they are, and complain when everything is going wrong. They manifest their lives, too, and are often angry, miserable and always feel like a victim.

A person who consciously creates their life tends to have an aura of positivity, peace, love and calm. They're clear about their vision, and even when they can't see the final outcome, they draw on reserves of faith and trust. People like to be around their energy. Regardless of what happens in their life, they look for the positives. Challenges become obstacles that require decision making, but do not bring the person to their knees.

The beauty of the conscious creator is that they make the world a better place, not just for themselves, of course, but *everyone around them*. It only takes a few minutes each day to transform your life. You know when you're becoming more conscious of how you create because all sorts of synchronicities start happening. Seeming coincidences become part of your daily life. They're affirmations from the Universe that you're on the right path. Consider this as spiritual grace. The more we live like this, the more readily and quickly our brain creates new neural pathways.

When you become fully aware that you, and you alone, are responsible for the state of your life, then everything around you will change. No longer will it be acceptable for you to blame other people or circumstances. You will also find that you won't wish to spend time with people who live in victim mode. You may become more aware of those who regularly start their sentences with "The problem is…"

Universe Wide Web

If you think the Internet is huge, imagine the energy behind the Universe Wide Web. We're constantly receiving and sending thoughts into it, and as a result either repel or attract those thoughts/emotions back into our life. We are vibrational magnets.

When spending time each day to consciously create, you can do so from the warmth and comfort of your cosy bed, or you can create a dedicated space in your home. Ensure the phone is off/down, and allow yourself to breathe deeply. Close your eyes. Let go of any fears, stresses or niggly worries. Fill your mind with a vision of how you would like your day to manifest. If you have a difficult meeting coming up, for example, see yourself filled with love and compassion for the other party, and a peaceful resolution. Use your mind like a cinema, and see beautiful pictures. Always envision the highest outcome. Experience the feeling of what you'd like to have happen in your day.

Empower yourself, one day at a time, by visualising the life you want. Start with today.

You, and only you, choose the thoughts that take up space in your head. Those that are based on love, optimism and gratitude, will trigger a completely different energy in every cell of your body (and life story) than those based on hate, anger, fear, jealousy, inadequacy and other negative feelings.

Heart Questions

What are the main thoughts that have residence in my head?
Do I find it easier to worry than to give thanks?
Do I take habitual 'comfort' in whingeing and complaining?
Do I actively participate in gossip, or do I refrain from feeding on the negative?
How do I respond to people in my inner circle who constantly complain?

This is no higher experience
for a human
than true,
heartfelt gratitude.

Conscious Intention

The simple truth is that we all have the ability to attract good, beautiful, life-changing and positive experiences and relationships into our lives. If you can envision a dream, then you can manifest it into your life. It all begins with a strong sense of desire. A fundamental law of the Universe is that *like attracts like*. I would say, first and foremost, that you have to have a willingness to suspend doubt, and to come from a place of wholehearted trust. To instigate and integrate change, it is essential that you recognise that you have a choice between being a victim or powerful conscious creator. Being willing to take 100% responsibility for your life is essential to creating the life of your dreams.

Manifestations In My Life
I want to share a few of the things I've manifested in my life, and how they came about. Mostly, it's because sometimes things come in ways we could never have imagined. The most important aspect to manifestation is to *trust* that the Universe will bring your desires to you, and not to bother questioning 'how' they'll arrive.

The standout manifestation in my life was attracting my soulmate, Paul. My experiences with men had not been great. I'd dated about fifty or so guys, and highly doubted that anyone could be right for me.

I was working at the Unity School of Metaphysics, and my boss, Reverend Graham Johnson, said to me "Veronika, you have to stop believing all men are bastards". He spoke gently and kindly, but his words seeped their way right down to the deepest part of my being. I wanted to say something like "but they are!", except, that in Graham, I had discovered a man who wasn't a bastard, and was indeed probably the first man I ever fully trusted. His words grew to life, and I changed my prevailing thought about the opposite sex to: *"Men are kind and wonderful"*.

I also wrote a list — a ridiculously long list — of the characteristics I wanted in my ideal man. Well, that was asking for trouble, wasn't it? What bloke could fit a few dozen specific requirements? I slept with that list under my pillow at night, reading it each day. I don't remember everything on the list now, but near the top were: kind, loving, vegetarian, humorous, sings to me, sensitive, spiritual…

That list was to change my life, not just because Paul walked through the door a few weeks later, but because I discovered the power of putting down one's desires in black and white. When Paul came into my life, I was engaged to a German chap called Peter. The relationship was strictly platonic. The engagement was to help him get residency in New Zealand. I was trying to be kind and helpful! (Don't shake your head in disgust, I thought I was doing a good deed!). Anyway, Peter and I had planned a housewarming and engagement party as we'd just rented a house together. He invited Paul along (he was Paul's masseur). The morning of the party, I said to Peter that I couldn't go through with the marriage. The party went ahead, but I remember looking over at

Paul and saying to my girlfriends "now that is a man I'd marry". Everything about Paul just felt so different to any man I'd ever met. But, he was nineteen years older than me. He couldn't possibly be interested.

Well, Peter moved out of the house, and my life, swiftly. I invited Paul for dinner, and he never went home again. We've been together for twenty-one years, and I swear I love that man more than is humanly possible.

Just before I met Paul, I was deeply involved in metaphysics, and was planning to travel to America to study and become a Minister of Metaphysics. The calling was so strong. However, it wasn't the only calling I could hear. In previous years, I was adamant I didn't want children. I'd been living in the UK, where I worked in animal welfare as a media officer. One night, I was awoken from a dream by a voice which said to me "You will write the Beautiful Birth book". I had no idea what this meant, but headed off the next morning to the local New Age bookshop around the corner from my modern studio flat in Hampshire. I was just browsing when two books literally fell of the shelf in front of me. How the heck does that actually happen? They were both books on waterbirths. I purchased them, and went home and devoured every page.

In no time at all, I was opening to the possibility of children. But what was particularly odd was that I felt a female child around me. Soon I was to hear her name, and receive pre-conception communication from her. So, by the time Paul showed up in my life (after me assuming I'd probably be a single mum because there were no men on the scene), I was pulled between my desire to study metaphysics full-time and that of having a daughter. When Paul came for dinner that sacred night which changed our lives forever, we played a game from Findhorn called The Transformation Game. We were both upfront about our desires, and our feelings for each other. We were manifesting at lightning speed.

By the way, the dream I had about the birth book was, I see in hindsight, a message about the book I wrote called *The Birthkeepers: reclaiming an ancient tradition*.

A couple of years after we'd got together, with a toddler and baby in tow, we had moved from New Zealand to Australia. Due to poor immigration advice (Paul being English, but a long-term New Zealand resident) we arrived in my homeland and found out he would not be allowed to work in the country. This caused quite a dilemma as I had two young breastfeeding children and didn't want to break that bond by going out to work. So we were on the bones of our bum, financially, for six months while deciding what to do. Returning to New Zealand wasn't really an option, work-wise, as that was the reason we'd left.

And then I had this bright idea that if we went to England, Paul would be able to work given he was, you know, English. There'd be no obstacles. One minor detail: we had NO money left.

However, when I get an idea in my head…

We started writing down what we wanted to manifest: living and working in England. It was a few weeks before Christmas, and a competition came on the local radio: 'sing us a Christmas carol and win $1,000 to be spent at the local shopping mall'.

Remember reading earlier that I wanted a man who would sing to me? The Universe must have had a chuckle when it read my list because Paul has a beautiful voice that he has made a career from in various ways, and is a professional singer. He pretended to be Luciano

Pavarotti, and did an amazing version of Silent Night. He won the competition, and believe it or not (though by now I hope you are a believer) the shopping mall had a travel agent! Tickets to the UK were booked! As I type these words, it is seventeen years ago to the day that we landed here on frozen English soil.

When I was a little girl, while my friends played happily with dolls, I was in the dirt pushing my Matchbox cars around, and building little neighbourhoods. I loved to drive! In my early twenties, I took a little sports car for a test drive along the New Zealand coastline around Auckland. Well, I didn't get that car from the showroom, but I did get a great husband and two kids! Clearly, a 2-seated sports car was not appropriate for that time in my life. Now, I'm the sort of girl who likes a simple life and isn't overly materialistic (though I do like beautiful items around me, and am not averse to comfort and luxury), but for some reason the desire to drive a convertible car never left me.

About a year ago, I saw a photo of a convertible and put it as a screen saver on my laptop. I just loved the shape of it, and figured that if I'm going to drive from A to B then I may as well do it in style rather than feeling like a rural hillbilly.

A few months later, a friend suggested I pop into a car yard and see what was there as I needed a car for my celebrant work. Well, that very model, in a different colour, was there. Happy dance! The weather was cold, but we put that top down and turned the heater on full, and drove through the beautiful Cumbrian countryside. Oh what fun! Money was otherwise engaged so I couldn't even put a deposit down. What I did do, though, was take a photo of the car and put it as the screen saver on my phone so I could see it every day.

Every time I saw that photo I thought "that car is soooo me!" I swear, it just had my name written all over it. The months went by, and nothing. I clicked onto the car dealer's website and couldn't believe it was still there. It must be a sign! I knew that the car would be mine. And then, a lump sum of money that was owed to me finally arrived. That gorgeous little car, albeit second hand and several years old, is such a pleasure to drive. I'm proud of myself for manifesting it! And what I love most is that it's real evidence for my daughters about the power of intention.

When Eliza was younger, she was desperate for us to get a Persian cat. She already had cats, and there was no need for any more. But my main reason for saying "no" was because I'd owned Persian cats in my early twenties, and let me tell ya, those little creatures are high maintenance. Even the boys! I didn't want to be stuck spending more time on grooming a cat than I do on myself! She spent ages on Google looking at Persians. She clearly hadn't registered any of my versions of 'no'. And then, months later, our friend, Jane, from the up the village, phoned and asked "Do you want another cat?" (Jane already had five, and couldn't take any more.) "He's a British short-haired Persian. He cost the owner £350 but you can have him for free. He's six months old, and needs a new home because the old cat where he lives isn't getting on with him."

I could not believe it. That daughter of mine manifested him right under my nose! A *short-haired* Persian, without the hairdressing requirements.

That cat, God love his furry self, has brought so much love and joy and laughter into our family over the past eight years. The power of intention. Don't leave home without it!

I also recently manifested a family holiday overseas. You can read more about that in the chapter called *I Create Adventure*.

Heart Questions

What are ten things you've manifested in your life, big or small, that have made you smile with the ease with which they showed up in your life?

How do you feel when people you know manifest good things into their life? Are you genuinely happy for them, or envious?

What do you experience when you're happy for other people's joys and successes?

Do you feel empowered or debilitated when you're jealous and envious of others?

*You are only ever
one thought away
from creating your day,
and manifesting
the life of your dreams.*

Decluttering

The Universe loves a vacuum! The quickest way to make changes in your life, and enhance your ability to manifest, is to get rid of items you no longer need, love or value. Set a goal of getting rid of *at least five things* a day for a week. And keep going! Charity shops welcome all sorts of items. Don't be afraid to let go of clothes, books, ornaments, shoes, CDs and so on. As you think about your future, and what you want to create for yourself, hold each item in your hand and ask yourself honestly (and without attachment) if it is part of your future life.

When releasing an item for the charity box, give thanks for how it has served you. Everything we own has a vibrational energy.

As a matter of course, I am in the habit of thanking items I use throughout the day: kettle, vacuum cleaner, woodstove, firewood, laptop, phones, clothesline, clothing, sofa, pillow, hair dryer, shower (especially when it's hot), car, washing machine, chopping knife, fridge, and so on. It takes but a second to wholeheartedly thank these items.

As someone who has moved countries several times, I'm pretty adept at narrowing my life down into a suitcase or two. But even though I've been settled now for seventeen years, I still love to declutter. It's freeing, and that sense of liberation creates huge internal shifts.

We hang onto so much, but none of us is taking anything with us when we leave the Earth. Nothing, that is, but love.

Heart Questions

When was the last time I decluttered?
How do I feel about letting go of: books, CDs and DVDs, ornaments, clothes?
Am I fearful of releasing items?
Why do I hang on to so many items?

Living in Alignment

As we embark on a life of conscious intention, there will be gifts along the way that show the Universe is listening to us. It may come in the form of a feather at your feet, or a rainbow, for example. Mostly you will notice amazing synchronicities happening in your life. Opportunities will show up, and you'll find yourself invited to events. PLEASE say yes to such opportunities if they feel good to you.

You'll notice a skip in your step, and a permanent sense of something wonderful about to happen. As the synchronicities increase, you'll become aware of really being in the right place at the right time, all of the time.

New people will come into your life, seemingly out of nowhere, and it will be like you've always known them. The connection will feel easy and beautiful. As your vibrations become higher, you may notice that you're way more sensitive to everything in the man-made environment. You might find yourself (possibly for the first time) declining alcohol or drugs, and you may find that you can't be around certain people any more.

You may struggle around radiation, such as that emitted from laptops, mobile phones, microwaves and so on. This is actually a positive thing! It shows your vibration is getting higher, and you'll feel a strong need to commune with Nature.

You will feel so expansive in your expression of gratitude. Complaining is the opposite of gratitude, and the more grateful you are the more aware you will become of anything negative around you, including words out of your mouth or those swimming in your head.

Repetition

As mentioned, I'm a member of our local gym, and the physical workouts have shown me a lot about the mind, too.

When you are developing muscles, you do repetitions of particular exercises, and then gradually build up your strength. When you start out, the weights are low, but over time you really see your strength and ability improving as you increase repetitions and weight.

The same idea applies to your manifestation muscles. At first, the idea of not complaining, for example, and of being grateful, can just seem like really hard work. Of course it does! We're in a culture which has a default setting of: whine, whine, whine; and is based on an adversarial system. Try not complaining for an hour. Rather than just give up and think it's too hard, commit to an hour of not complaining (about anything). Then try two hours. If you're reluctant to try this, perhaps it's worth asking yourself why you're so invested in complaining. What are the benefits of it?

With gratitude, the easiest way to start is by keeping a gratitude journal and writing down five things each day that you're grateful for. This is a beautiful ritual to do just before you go to sleep at night.

There was a time in our life when we were struggling,

financially, for about six months. But if you were to have read my gratitude journal from that time, you'd have had no inclination of the hardship. The Universe gifted us with so much love, joy, friendship, boxes of tropical fruit, and gorgeous gifts. The more grateful I became, the more I received.

When you're in the habit of writing your gratitude list, why not also say it out loud? As you do this, really feel the overwhelming appreciation opening your heart. This is no higher experience for a human than true, heartfelt gratitude.

As you start to become a regular manifestor, I recommend writing all your affirmations (in the present tense) beginning with the words: *I am grateful...*

Wok around the Clock

The first time after I'd travelled to England, I went back to New Zealand with about $10 to my name, and no job. Nothing new there! For some reason this was my pattern around landing in foreign countries. Anyway, I arrived in beautiful New Zealand, and within about twenty-four hours someone offered me a job. It was in a jigsaw-puzzle factory on the assembly line (BORING!), but I was grateful for the income because it meant I could get a flat. I set to writing a list of things I'd need. Wok, table, mirror...and so the list went on. No one knew about my list, but within a day someone asked me if I wanted a wok and a table. Now, I know I'm good at manifesting, but the speed with which these small items turned up astounded even me. I've often had a thought, such as: I need a briefcase; and right out of the blue someone gives me the very thing I'm wanting. This has happened throughout my life.

So, manifesting isn't just about the big things or

experiences. It's anything and everything. It may be physical items, and it may be experiences, relationships and emotional states. In the end, once you come to really understand your ability to create, you realise that you're like a magician able to conjure at will.

Heart Questions

Have I noticed signs from the Universe that I'm in alignment with my values and my soul purpose?
In what ways have I seen affirmations from the Universe?

The future changes
with every choice
we make.

Living in Divine Harmony

This book is now divided into twelve themes based on the astrological houses in the birth chart. The houses cover each area of human life. As a second-generation astrologer, I have come to see that these are universal human stories we all experience to one degree or another. To me, it makes sense to explore these topics when consciously creating our life.

You don't have to believe or understand astrology in any way to benefit from this. The experiences of each house are merely a guide so that you can create a fuller picture of the human experience, and bring consciousness to the topics.

Many people believe we are victims of Fate, and that we're puppets on a string. It is true that some people have more than their share of upheaval, grief and trauma to deal with. On the surface, it can seem that some have blessed lives while others appear to always be at war with life itself. Is it possible to change our lives so profoundly as to be empowered, rather than victimised, regardless or *in spite of* what comes our way? I believe so.

Some of the happiest and most vibrant people I know have had true tragedies and heartbreak in their lives. Their attitude, however, has enabled them to keep enjoying their human existence.

The ultimate act of spirituality is consciously creating your life, rather than being a victim of fate. As you become skilled at creating your day, you won't need to refer to these sections. Initially, though, it is worth going through them as a way of seeing how much balance there is between them in your life.

"Surround yourself with people who are only going to lift you higher."
~ **Oprah**

Appearance

I Create My Identity

I am, therefore I am

When we come into this world, we quickly develop a self-image based on how we were greeted at birth (that threshold between Spiritside and Earthside). Our personality is, in essence, a 'defence mechanism' against/towards the world.

Let's explore the themes of body, self-awareness and identity, for this is about how we appear to others, and the happier we are within our skin, the more easily we're able to function in this world.

Understanding and developing your individuality, and what you look like, all come under this theme of appearance. This astrological house describes where and how we project ourselves onto other people, and it includes many aspects of our demeanour, manners, and physical attributes or disabilities. This is where people register their first impressions about us: Are we shy? Abrupt? Friendly? Beautiful? Considerate? Sexy? Sophisticated? Hurried? Slow? Chatty? Self-centred? Self-aware? Withdrawn? A Show Pony? Pedantic? Businesslike? Eccentric? Dreamy? Of course, as humans, we're complex and have many different facets to our personality.

Our physical appearance is a bit like looking at the front door of a house. It's the first thing people see when they come to our home, but it doesn't show all the rooms inside. The front door lets people know whether they're welcome inside (to get to know you better) or not. What they see — that first impression — may not be what they get if they hang around.

When we make the conscious decision to start creating our day, some of the questions that come up will be about how to become the highest version of ourselves. We can do this by asking:

Who am I?

How do I present myself to the world?

In what way do I value my body, particularly my head and face?

Is my physical body a representation of my personality? Does it mirror my approach to life?

Consider your vitality, weight, how you approach life, and the way you interact with others, especially strangers.

In some ways, you might think that you have no 'say' over how you look. How you *present* yourself, though, is something you can become conscious of and work with, if necessary. The more alive and vital we feel, the more this shines from us.

When you were born, you arrived Earthside and immediately had a reaction to this life. Your body responded in ways which helped you adapt. It may have withdrawn, or been excited about the new adventure. Maybe you became secretive. Your body reflected the impressions you had of the world (whether they were true or not), and the ones the world (family, in particular) had of you.

When I was four or five, we had some neighbours whose company I enjoyed. They were an elderly, childless, Eastern European couple called Blanka and Lotzi. They took great pleasure in telling me how beautiful I was. For some reason, I always felt uncomfortable about it, as if it couldn't possibly be true. How is it that even as a young child we can already feel insecure about our body and our looks? I look back on a photo of me at that age and think "What a cutie! I was totally adorable." I can see what they saw.

As a parent, I told my daughters every day how beautiful they were to me, and yet, sure enough, somewhere along the way they received other messages and my words were dismissed.

Loving ourselves isn't egotistical, but essential for developing and maintaining a healthy sense of self-value.

If your body is a place where you feel repulsion, and you dislike touch or looking at yourself, consider a flower essence to help reach the core wound.

Australian Bush Flower Essences
Billy Goat Plum, Five Corners, Mulla Mulla, and Wisteria. Or try **Bach's**: Crab Apple.

Creating your day will involve finding ways to really nurture your physical body (regardless of what shape it currently is in).

Physically, here are some ways to energise your body:

[] Rebounding (mini trampoline). This works every muscle in the body, and is gentle on the knees and suitable for all levels of fitness.

[] Yoga or Pilates, dancing, walking, skipping, running, weight-resistance exercises, swimming.

Music
Drums are particular effective for enlivening the physical body. Listen to music with a strong beat.

Aromatherapy
Identify scents which appeal to you, and incorporate them into your daily life. My favourites include eucalyptus, jasmine, coconut, ginger and lemongrass. Great scents for honouring the physical body include cinnamon, sandalwood, cedar wood and lavender. Massage this combination into your skin: Pink grapefruit, sweet orange and black pepper.

Gemstones
Try wearing black tourmaline or onyx.

Meditation and Visualisation Image
Use the image of a front door to help you establish your sense of self. Through meditation or visualisation, create a front door that is symbolic of how you would like to present yourself to the world. What type of door represents who you would like to be seen as? For example, is it hidden away behind a hedge? What colour is it? Does it have an electronic doorbell or an

old-fashioned bell? Are there plants beside the door? Is there a welcome mat? Is the door made of wood or glass? Perhaps the door is, in fact, two doors which open wide? Create a door symbolic of you and the energy you give out when you first meet people.

Healing Modalities

Develop your leadership skills, primal-scream therapy, rebirthing, dance, sports, mirror work, cranial osteopathy, running, weight-resistance training, Indian head massage.

Mirror Work

If affirming that you love or value yourself feels alien, try standing in front of a mirror (ideally naked, but do it with clothes on as a first step) and looking in your eyes (lovingly!) as you retrain your body and mind with new messages.

This is such a brilliant way of learning to love yourself, especially if you weren't validated as a child. Yes, it may feel odd or uncomfortable when you first start, but persist. Be kind to yourself. You may feel angry the first few times, but that's a normal response to years of feeling inadequate. But please, persist, because mirror work is the number-one choice of healing modality for developing self-awareness, respect and love.

Affirmations

I am aware of how I move and act.
I am beautiful and attractive.
I am dynamic.
I am wonderful.
I love myself.
I nurture my body through eating nourishing foods.

I take care of my body by exercising regularly.
I live, move, and have my being in (grace, beauty, love, etc).
I am taking good care of myself.
I am aware that I attract life's experiences to me.
I have a strong sense of self.
I am aware of my body's boundary.

Heart Questions
How do I feel about my physical body?
Am I aware of mannerisms?
Do I feel comfortable in my own skin?
In what ways could I improve my sense of body and movement?
What do I feel when I look in the mirror? Am I kind to myself or do I speak unkindly?
Do I smile or scowl as an instinctive response to strangers?
Do I have a strong sense of my body so that I am not violated by others?

Acquisition

I Create My Values

I have, therefore I am

When we enter this life, we start with an awareness of
our body. Were we met by gentle hands and soft voices?
Were we cut from our mother's womb? Did cold, hard,
steel forceps squeeze our head and drag us down the
birth canal? Was our mother drugged?

Did we leave the darkish womb and enter a room
lit with fluorescent lights and the air smelling of
disinfectant? Or, perhaps, we were born by candlelight
in a warm birthing pool in our parents' home, and
welcomed in peace and love and gratitude?

Do we like being held snugly? Are we wrapped
warmly enough? Are we fed when we're hungry? Can
we hear mother's heartbeat? (The same one we heard
for nine months in the womb.) Did we find comfort

through her soft, malleable breasts, or we were we fed from a bottle? These initial impressions shape us, and influence our personality long before we can verbalise our opinions.

By the time we have a good sense of our body, and that we own it (therefore, are separate from Mum), we then move onto an awareness of *what* we own, and what brings us pleasure. Ideally, we'd still be breastfeeding, but generally by toddlerhood we're eating other foods, too. Our taste buds come alive with a variety of flavours. The world around us takes on new meaning. We discover food in all its forms, and we appreciate music, and can determine whether something is ugly or beautiful to us.

We develop the capacity to say "NO!" or "Mine!" We understand our desires, and we either want more of something or don't want it at all.

Many parents fear this part of parenting, and yet when we honour a child's desire as to what brings him or her pleasure, then we're allowing them to develop in a way that's true to them, rather than us. Why force a child to eat chicken if he prefers watermelon? Why put your child in an itchy synthetic dress if she prefers a natural fabric? Obviously, as parents, there are times when we have to set boundaries, and there may be a conflict of wills. Perhaps, however, it is the very curtailment of what we desire that shuts us down in later life when making claims on what we value or want.

The toddler years (when we define our values) are primal and sensual. Could it be because so many adults are removed from what they truly desire that they find the toddler years of their children to be 'troublesome'.

The desire part of our life is instinctual. Intellect doesn't come into this realm (hence the inability to

68

reason with a toddler). Our basic wants and needs stem from thirst, hunger, comfort and warmth. We begin with basic desires and needs, then to wants, and then move onto the more abstract form of values.

If you have trouble identifying your needs, wants and desires, then it's likely that you weren't nurtured in a way that suited you during your early childhood, particularly around food. Later in life, this manifests in how we approach money, what we own, and our self-worth. In short, this part of life is to do with how we acquire comfort and material security.

Money
Love it, or hate it…it's unlikely you can ignore money unless you're part of an undiscovered tribe in the Amazonian rainforests. Wealth is more than money in the bank, or vast swathes of real estate. True wealth is to do with self-worth. As we create our day, understanding our values — including what it is about ourselves that we appreciate — makes a huge difference to every other part of our life.

"Poverty hides itself in thought,
before it surrenders to purses."
~ Kahlil Gibran

Have a look at the following list of values. What are your top three? Please note that one isn't better than the other, nor is it a comprehensive list. What's important is to recognise what has resonance with you, and then look at how you incorporate that in your life. How much 'value' do you give your values? Does your life accurately reflect them?

Accountability
Achievement
Adventure
Beauty
Community
Creativity
Discipline
Efficiency
Excellency
Excitement
Faith
Freedom
Friendship
Fun
Goodness
Hard work
Harmony
Hope
Independence
Individuality
Integrity
Justice
Love
Loyalty
Meaning
Openness

Personal Growth
Practicality
Privacy
Reliability
Resilience
Resourcefulness
Respect
Security
Self-reliance
Self-respect
Service
Simplicity
Success
Sustainability
Tolerance
Trust
Truth
Wisdom

My top three values are beauty, integrity and simplicity. There are many more I could choose, but these are the ones I couldn't be without.

How do your values relate to money and security? Are they connected?

In my life, abundance is reflected in the way my values shape my day. For example, I thrive when there is beauty in my home, such as fresh flowers, large pot plants, incense burning, beeswax candles lit, and gorgeous music playing. And I love it when the place is clean and tidy. It's not about having it that way for other people, but for me. I value the simplicity of hanging my washing outside to dry, or having dry wood by the woodstove. My meals are cooked from scratch using fresh fruit and vegetables, and unprocessed wholefoods.

The way we do money
is the way we do life

I veer towards simplicity, and do believe that less is more.

I value living with integrity, and having friends who share this value. In my life, my close friendships are with people who share the core ingredients of integrity: honesty, kindness, reliability, and a strong moral compass. I value people who stand by their principles no matter what, and are secure in who they are. These are the people who are the same in company as when no one is watching.

What we value, is what we tend to accumulate, and what our resources are. Essentially, it's about how many, and what sort of, toys we have in our toy box!

Our values should also include our skills or innate gifts, as these are a precious resource. If our world stopped using money as a currency, what skills do you have that you could barter for food and other life essentials?

How do you register your self-worth? Ask yourself: how good do I feel about who I am? (This is different to our personality, or what we look like, or the impression we give to others.) This is really a question of *Do I love myself?* If not, why not?

Do I enjoy my own company? If not, why not?

Do I have a strong enough boundary to say "no" to others so that I can say "yes" to myself? If not, why not?

When we come to see that we are our greatest resource, then enormous attitudinal healing towards our values, and a new consciousness towards money, can take place. It is said that the way we do money is the way we do life. How does that statement feel to you? Can you see the parallel?

I am often at my happiest when pottering in the garden in the vegetable patch on a deliciously sunny day, or chopping fresh fruit and vegetables in the kitchen. These are active ways of integrating the energies of acquisition. A well-stocked pantry is another. I love seeing my glass Kilner jars stocked with seeds, nuts, beans and pulses. It gives me a feeling of abundance equal to seeing my blueberry bushes heaving with ripe berries, or the fridge filled with vegetables.

Regularly inspect your finances and become *conscious* of all income and outgoings. This stimulates your money psychology, and will make you more proactive about what you bring into your life.

"What we gonna do when the money runs out?"

When my girls were young, a friend leant me a CD by the singer David Gray. There was a song I sang along to called *What We Gonna Do When the Money Runs Out?* I enjoyed David Gray, but one day one of my daughters turned to me, a worried look on her face, and asked "What *are* we going to do when the money runs out, Mummy?" Oh my goddess, what a wake-up call! I stopped listening to that CD immediately, and became a heck of a lot more conscious about the lyrics of songs I listened to (especially when my children were around).

Investments

Your three primary investments will ideally include: yourself, the present, the future.

In what ways do you invest in yourself? Perhaps it is through education, or buying books to self-study? Maybe you invest in your health by exercising every day and avoiding all forms of sugar. Is it possible you invest in yourself by having regular haircuts or massages?

Consider the ways in which you invest. Do you invest *time* so that you aren't rushing about all hours of the day? Do you invest in *silence* so that your brain can come to a place of equilibrium? Do you accept compliments? Do you take time to appreciate what other people bring into your world?

How do you invest in your present life? What are you doing to provide comfort for yourself?

What future investments do you make? Perhaps you have a private pension fund. Maybe you invest in your future by making choices now that will allow you freedom and independence later on.

What are your top five ways of investing in yourself?
1.
2.
3.
4.
5.

What are five ways you're investing in the present?
1.
2.
3.
4.
5.

How are you investing in the future?
1.
2.
3.
4.
5.

Energising your values
Choose your top three values from the list on page 70.

1.
2.
3.

How do they play out in your life?
Why do you bestow such meaning on them?
Can you use them in any way to earn an income?
How do they nourish you?
In what ways can you utilise them to create your day?

Money Magic
Need to manifest money? Find a money note, and breathe it in. We all have a "money consciousness" which can be activated in the brain. As the smell of the note enters your being, tell yourself:

I love money, it helps me pay the bills.
I love money, it allows me to buy new clothes.
I love money, it feeds my family.
I love money, it smells great!
I love money, it allows me to help others.
I love money, it allows me to make the world a better place.
I love money, it fills my bank account.
I love money, it allows me to travel.
I love money, it allows me to live luxuriously.
I love money, and I let it flow into my life.

Make a commitment, today, to change how you view money (if you need to). Consider it your ally, in that it will allow you to create a better world. Decide on how much money you want to regularly come into your life, and then set the ball of intention rolling. As you create your day, be clear about your income and that it will *always* be greater than your outgoings.

Some people repel abundance in financial form. Let's be clear: having more money will not change who you are, but will amplify what is important to you and your fundamental values.

Make a Money Tree

My Dad, who frankly made a lot of money in his lifetime, left me the unfortunate legacy of telling me that money doesn't grow on trees. Boy it's taken some work to let go of that stupid belief. Money *does* grow on trees. Money comes from trees! Here's an idea you might like to try: start sticking paper money notes to a house plant or a large wooden branch, until the whole thing looks like a money tree. That will shift your money vibration big time. Keep your money tree visible.

Money and Bills

LOVE your bills. Show gratitude for them, because they show you that the creditor trusts your ability to pay. Be thankful every time you receive an invoice, and every time you make a payment.

Money Plants

Have you ever noticed those funny-looking plants in a Chinese takeaway? They're called money plants. If you find them in a florist or garden centre, grab two, and place one at your front door to invite money in, and one at your back to keep money circulating in your life.

Mindful Manifestation Ritual

Each day, I create a ritualistic atmosphere: I light incense, and play a chant called *Om Namah Shivaya*. In this sacred space, I write an affirmation fifty-five times. I do this for five days in a row, then begin a new affirmation.

I write my affirmations in the present tense, always using positive words, and begin each sentence with the words *I am grateful…*

Manifestation Chant

To chant *Om Namah Shivaya* bestows deep spiritual experiences, and even gifts one with supernatural abilities when practised deeply and correctly. The meaning is this:

Om Before there was a Universe, there was a vibrationless void of pure existence. From this, came the vibration which started the Universe: *Om* (Aum), the sacred and primordial sound.

Namah means 'to bow'.

Shivaya refers to Shiva, but it also means 'inner self'. So, to understand and experience properly, Om Namah Shivaya means *"I bow to the inner Self."*

Regular practice of this will bring you closer to your divine nature. It awakens one to a higher consciousness. The five holy vowels represent the seed sounds of the five elements of creation: earth, water, fire, air and ether. An alternative translation is: *"May the greatest that can be in this world be created within myself, within others, and within the world"*.

I've long been a believer and practioner of affirmations. However, this 5 days x 55 ritual is

Having more money
will not change who you are,
but will amplify
what is important to you,
and your fundamental values.

particularly powerful. I highly recommend Sarah Prout's Ancient Manifestation Ritual: sarahprout.com

Prayer to the Goddess Abundantia
"Help me replace my money fears with a sense of openness and trust. Show me how to be grateful for everything in my life. Share your abundance with me."

Affirmations
I create a new attitude to my values.
I actively live my values.
I am conscious of how I earn and spend my money.
I am deliberately receiving new avenues of income.
I am worthy.
I am a child of the Universe. I have a right to be here.
I expect the best.
I create delicious meals for myself and others.
I am open to discovering new values.
I have everything I need.
I am a magnet for divine prosperity.
I love and bless my current income.
I deserve to prosper.
There is plenty for everyone, including me.
I deserve to have and enjoy nice things.
I focus on what is of true value to me.
I attract what I value.
I have enough.
I am enough.
I am prosperous.
Abundance is mine.
I am grateful for my income.
I am open to new avenues of income.
My income is constantly increasing.
I am skilled at...

My gifts are…
I am a magnet for money.
I am worthy of enjoying pleasure.

Aromatherapy
Sweet orange and lime

Flower Essences
Abund (Australian Bush Flower Essences)
Positive Flow aura spray (Healing Orchid Essences)
Go Create (Alaskan Flower Essence) is an abundance formula to clear limiting beliefs.

Wild Rose, Chestnut Bud, Chicory, Iris, Tansy, Corn, Nasturtium, Gentian.

Healing Modalities
Shiatsu, massage, good-quality chocolate, sound therapy, saving money. Singing activates the acquisition energy. Humming or chanting works well, too.

Allow Pleasure In Your Day
Eat delicious food, slowly, savouring each mouthful
Smell the flowers
Sleep on clean sheets
Walk barefoot on the grass
Watch the stars
Marvel at the moonlight
Make popcorn using organic coconut oil
Close your eyes and listen to beautiful music
Feel sunlight on your skin
Clean your home using only 100%-pure essential oils

In the end, all the money we seek to acquire in life is for the purpose of creating *pleasure or material security*. Define your pleasures (with or without money), and see what has meaning to you. What delights your soul? What forms of pleasure make you feel glad to be alive? How often do you let them into your life? I've met people who seem miffed by the idea of what brings them pleasure. Here's a list of some of my favourite things. Maybe it will inspire you.

I love...
Thunder and lightning
Sun-ripened mangos
Cuddling new babies
Hot sunshine
Starlight
Laughter
Waking up to birdsong
Listening to Strauss waltzes
Chatting with people I love
Ceremonies
Butterflies
Seasons
Being massaged
Sleeping in
Getting up early
Flowers
Making love
Walking barefoot on grass
The way my husband makes me coffee
Swimming
Reading
Writing
Playing

Beeswax candles
Sitting on moss
Walking in a forest on my own
Lying on the grass and being held by Mother Earth
Smiles
My family
Heartfelt connections with others
Home cooking
Cuddling with my husband (or daughters) on the sofa

Meditation or Visualisation Image
Use the image of a children's toy box to help you establish your sense of what you value. Through meditation or visualisation, imagine this box filled with everything that brings you pleasure and security, including nourishing food, beautiful clothing, houses, property, skills, talents, and money. As you mentally place items in there, or take them out to play with, give thanks for them.

Heart Questions

Do I love money?
Do I feel worthy of abundance?
Does money come easily into my life?
How do I feel about food? Is it a source of pleasure?
Am I open to new avenues of abundance, or do I believe it can only come through my job?
What are my skills and talents?
Do I regularly allow myself to have pleasure? Do I feel guilty when I have an enjoyable experience?
Is money a struggle?
Am I always hanging out till pay day or benefit-payments day?
Am I generous with my money (and time)?

Do I save for a rainy day or trust there won't be rainy days?
Do I give away money (and time) too readily?
Do I have strong boundaries around money that I loan to friends and family?
Are people always coming to me for money?
Do I fear money?

Communication

I Create My Voice

I think, therefore I am

When I was a young child, my mother often sent me to the neighbours to hang out with them because her ears got sore from all my talking! Who knew I'd grow up to be a writer and public speaker? These days, I talk less and listen more. A lot of my communication is through the written word, but as a five-year-old I didn't have that facility, so I talked. A lot.

This area of life is vital to making our way with ease in the world. It's not just about how we communicate with our siblings, neighbours, lover or children, but how we speak or write to those in the wider world. Do we feel hampered? Are we scared to speak in case we say the wrong thing? Are we guilty of over-talking and not listening? Perhaps we always feel the weight of our words?

We covered appearance and body mannerisms earlier, and while most of our communication (about 80%) is through body language (hence the importance of body awareness), those words that we do speak need to be clear, articulate and delivered with care in order to be received as effectively as possible.

Activating the Voice

Talk to yourself in front of a mirror and get a sense of how you come across. Do you mumble? Do you cover your mouth while speaking? Do you look up at the ceiling when you talk, rather than into the other person's eyes?

Effective communication can be learned by children and adults. It's never too late. It is easy to think that it is something that you'd only need if you were working in a corporate environment, but these skills are just as important to all of us. How often do you come up against situations where you need to communicate clearly?

Learning the basics of assertiveness training will stand you in good stead for life. It's about learning the balance between aggressiveness (bullying and intimidation) and passiveness (or victimhood/martyrdom). It is human nature to swing from one extreme to the other from time to time, but with practice you can find yourself more stable in how you choose to communicate. When we find ourselves veering towards one extreme or the other, we can be sure that we're not communicating effectively. Being assertive is always a balanced response.

When we master the art of being assertive, we learn to feel better about who we are. In short, our confidence and self-esteem improve. So, interestingly, the more confident we become as communicators, the more readily and easily we'll attract acquisition in our lives.

If we find ourselves feeling inadequate, regretful or

guilty, we need to acknowledge that we're behaving in a passive way. On the other hand, if we find ourselves feeling critical or angry during a conversation, this might be an indication of aggressive behaviour or tendencies on our part.

Here is what I have found useful when communicating with people who are being manipulative or aggressive towards me. One response would be to mirror their behaviour and yell back, but if I can come from a consciously chosen calm place, and use words which are not defensive, but instead placate the aggressor, then it allows me to meet them without agreeing to their demands or bullying. Sometimes this approach may involve agreeing with some of the points the aggressor is making, and by doing so the other person suddenly (and unexpectedly) feels less confrontational. In a short

An assertive person recognises the other as his equal.

period of time, I usually find that they have calmed down and a proper conversation can begin. This way of communicating is known as 'fogging' because what it does is create a wall of fog in which arguments are placed but not returned.

Another technique involves an assertiveness skill known as calm persistence. It requires you to repeat what you want, over and over, without raising the tone of your voice, or changing the subject, or becoming irritated or angry. By repeating your request, it ensures that the conversation doesn't become an argument. You need to stay calm, be clear in what you're asking for, and not get sidetracked by other issues. This technique is particularly effective when needing to return faulty goods.

Perhaps the most important aspect of being assertive lies in being able to own and express your feelings. For example, rather than saying to your husband "You make me so angry!", you could say: "I feel angry when you leave dirty dishes in the sink". It removes blame, and as soon as we take away finger-pointing then the situation is ours. We *own* our feelings, and our perception.

Being assertive means, amongst other things, being able to say 'no' without feeling guilty. For example,

*"If we were supposed to talk
more than we listen,
we would have two tongues and one ear."*
~ Mark Twain

your partner wants you to spend Christmas with the in-laws, which is your personal version of hell. Once you begin learning to say no to others (which by the very notion of it, means saying YES to yourself) it becomes easier. You soon learn that you don't even have to offer an excuse. You could offer an explanation: "I really love Christmas, and I really love you. I need to have our own Christmas, just us two and the baby. I feel exhausted after the birth. This is a special time for the family that you and I have made together. Perhaps you could visit your parents on Boxing Day?" There's a difference between an explanation and an excuse, and you'll learn that you're not obliged to give either.

Women, in particular, are experts at having their precious time sucked up by anyone and everyone. By learning to be assertive, you become a guardian as to how and where you spend your time. You develop healthy boundaries, and set limits with grace, ease and self respect.

Many people feel that by becoming assertive, others around them won't like them anymore, or think they're being selfish. Assertive people don't make others uncomfortable. Passive and aggressive people do.

Key points to remember as you develop your assertive voice, include:
[] keep your voice calm, even if you're angry
[] breathe deeply to steady yourself
[] make eye contact
[] stick to the point, and don't bring up unnecessary topics
[] don't apologise if you haven't done anything wrong
[] be polite.

In the beginning, you might find it really uncomfortable being assertive, especially if you're not used to recognising what you need or feel.

A needy or manipulative person may even try to label you as aggressive or arrogant, but an assertive person is neither of those things. When you become skilled at this way of communicating, you'll find that neither you nor the person you're addressing feels abused or upset or invalidated.

An arrogant person feels superior. A passive person feels like a victim. An assertive person recognises the other as his equal.

A passive person communicates through hinting, or making noises, such as sighing, and hoping someone will take notice. They don't openly ask for what they need.

An aggressive person uses intimidation to get their message across. They might also use sarcasm, yelling or other methods of bullying.

An assertive person asks for what they need, and they own their communication. They are mindful about respecting other people's opinions. They consciously ensure their body and facial language is relaxed. This confidence spills over into other areas of their life.

When developing the art and skill of assertiveness, stick to your own feelings, rather than blaming. Avoid making assumptions about the other person's behaviour.

Learn to ask for what you need. For example: "I feel scared when you yell at our daughter. I would feel more comfortable if you spoke to her gently".

"I feel sad when you come home from work and go straight to the TV without asking me how my day was. I feel more connected and able to be intimate with you when you've interacted with me and the children."

An assertive person checks in with their own feelings, and knows their own limits.

Learning to Listen

According to research, we only remember about 25% to 50% of what we hear. This is because we don't actively listen. Many conflicts and misunderstandings occur because of this. Remedying the way we listen is just as important in the home as it is in the workplace and wider world. There are four things we experience when we actively listen: we *gather information*; we *learn*; we can *enjoy*; and hopefully, we *understand*. To become an effective communicator means developing a high level of self-awareness. Once you come to understand (and enhance) your personal way of communicating, you'll develop a lifelong way of creating good relationships with other people.

To develop and build active-listening skills, you must learn to really listen. It requires hearing more than just the words which are being spoken, but the underlying messages. You begin to do this by not allowing yourself to be distracted by anything else or by forming counter-arguments in your head as the other person is speaking. If you find yourself becoming bored, it *may* mean that you're not listening properly. One way to help yourself stay tuned in to the speaker is to quietly repeat their words in your head. (This works well for remembering names, too.)

If you've ever been talking to someone and felt like you weren't being heard, you'll know how devaluing it is to your self-esteem. Acknowledge the person as they speak, by nodding your head or saying yes, or if appropriate, a gentle touch on the hand or arm (for example, when someone is sad). This is true heart-to-heart communication. Although you're not talking (because you're listening), your body can talk. It can say "yes, I hear you". With practice and experience, you'll come to naturally find the times and appropriate places to interject with a comment or a question.

Non-verbal communication is powerful. Look at the person who is talking to you, and avoid letting yourself be distracted by whatever is happening in the environment. Avoid doing anything while they're talking. Don't plan conversations in your head. Just listen. Pay attention to their body language. Eighty percent of what we communicate comes via the rest of the body. As you actively listen, make sure that your posture is open and accommodating.

We all have judgements and assumptions bubbling just below the surface, and they can distort what we filter through our ears. In order to avoid this happening, you may need to repeat what you've heard (or think you've heard) by saying "What I'm hearing is that..."

If you're still unclear, you can say "So what you mean is...?"

Always allow someone to finish speaking before you respond. As parents, we are modelling respect and understanding when we actively listen to someone. Our children witness us as we gain information and perspective by being honest, open, and asserting ourselves respectfully.

Humans are creatures of habit, but even if you've had forty years of ineffective communication, there is no reason why you can't learn to be assertive and become an active listener. If you set yourself a goal to truly hear what another person is saying, then you'll find yourself beginning to communicate in ways which are authentic, deliberate and open. Learning to ask questions, deflecting, and paraphrasing are important communication tools which can be learnt by anyone who truly desires to hear and to be heard.

Effective listening skills are at the heart of all positive human relationships, and form a firm and loving foundation in harmonious family life.

Hearing is about sounds, while listening is about what you focus on. It means paying attention, not just to the words you hear, but to the body language, the tone, and being receptive to everything the person is communicating. On a personal level, all of our social interactions improve. Focus on the speaker, not on anything else. Make eye contact. Be truly present. This is the same whether you're communicating with children or adults.

The more we can live and breathe assertiveness and active listening, the better a role model we become for our children and the adults around us. It isn't something you learn in a weekend, but can take a lifetime to refine. There are no downsides to becoming and being an effective listener and an assertive person.

Effective listening skills
are at the heart
of all positive human relationships,
and form a firm and loving foundation
in harmonious family life.

Ways to use and improve your voice and communication

Practising any sort of sound or movement from your mouth will start to activate the communication energy. Try whistling, chanting, humming and singing. If you're feeling confident enough, join a choir or see a voice coach. Learn to clearly enunciate your consonants.

As you go through your day, let your mouth be expressive. Laugh, yawn, kiss.

Sing when you're doing housework, gardening, cooking, driving and exercising.

Write a letter. Keep a journal. Write to-do lists.

Be a conscious speaker, and a conscious listener. One of the things I'm challenged by, is when I'm chatting with someone on the phone and I can hear them tapping away at the keyboard, or they're also having a conversation with someone in the room. Be 100% present in all your communications. If you can't talk/listen at that moment, then respect yourself and the other person enough to say so. This is one area of life where multitasking is not of benefit.

In our culture, so much time and money is spent on what we look like, and next to no effort is given to what we sound like. Record your voice and become familiar with how you sound.

Gemstones

Turquoise, Sodalite, Amazonite Chrysocola, Lapis, Blue Opal. Choose one to wear around your neck.

Flower Essences
Cosmos
To enable: integration of ideas and speech; coherent thinking; mercurial expression.

Trumpet Vine
To enable: articulation and colour in verbal expression; active, dynamic projection of oneself in social situations.

Cerato
To help you to speak your truth.

Healing Modalities
Drink more water
Read in front of the mirror
Singing
Record your voice. Consider a voice coach.
Write letters
Start a blog
Write a novel
Speak up

Affirmations
It is safe for me to speak my truth.
I am articulate.
I am a clear communicator.
I speak with love.
I trust my voice.
I listen to my ideas.
It is safe for me to speak.
My messages and language are comfortably received.
I am curious.

Aromatherapy
Pink grapefruit and tangerine. Also, sage and eucalyptus.

Meditation and Visualisation Image
In your mind, imagine a large classroom chalkboard to symbolise learning and communication. What does it say on there? Is this something you can articulate? Use this image to bring you answers to questions.

Heart Questions
How comfortable am I about speaking to others?
Do I feel strong in my voice?
Was I listened to as a child?
Do I actively listen to others?
How do I express myself in the written word?

In 2012, researchers from the Albert Einstein College of Medicine found that being optimistic played a major role in living a long life.

"Thoughts become things.
If you see it in your mind,
you will hold it in your hand."
~ Bob Proctor

Security

I Create My Home

I feel, therefore I am

From my small, colourful, hand-woven round African basket, I pick up sticks of incense. I light each one with a match, my eyes resting in the flicker of the flame before blowing out the small fire: and then I place the sticks around my home. Instantly, I feel a sense of calm. I rest the incense in the large pots which hold luscious houseplants. Mozart plays quietly on the stereo. I am at peace. I am home.

Home is our foundation, even if we work 18-hour days. It is the place we come to undress from the world. To consciously make your home a happy place means that you always have a strong foundation, or sense of security, to your life. Home is a container for all our emotions. If walls could talk, hey?

What changes a house into a home? Why do some

dwellings make you feel instantly at ease, while others have you looking for the nearest exit? On a surface level, it may have to do with cleanliness and orderliness, but it goes deeper than that. Our home speaks of who we are. Do we invest in sacred space by only having those things around us which have meaning? Are we hoarders? Do we take note of our surroundings?

For me, home is a sanctuary, and I adorn it with beeswax candles, fresh colourful flowers, healing crystals, art and photos which have meaning, nurturing music, supportive companionship, and healthy indoor plants.

Astrologically, the fourth house is not just about home, but our deepest feelings, the subconscious, and our ancestry. The most southern point of the birth chart is known as the midnight hour. This area of human life is like an artesian basin (underground lake) filled with our deepest, unspoken memories, and DNA passed down the family line. Some people use the energy of this area of human life to really study the family tree and to connect the dots of the archetypes which continue with each generation. In the second house of astrology, we learnt about material security. In the fourth house, we (hopefully) experience emotional security.

On a more mundane level, but every bit as meaningful, is making a study of your home. As your base of operations, what can you do to make your living space a comfy and cosy nest?

Kitchen
This is the heart of the home in so many ways. We come here to prepare nourishing foods and beverages, and to feed ourselves and our loved ones.

When you create your day, consider your kitchen as a

vital heartbeat to your well-being. Is it welcoming? Why not display baskets of fresh fruit or root vegetables? Perhaps there is a large Kilner glass dispenser for containing fresh water with lemon slices and mint leaves. Maybe you have a devotional altar to bring mindfulness as you begin crafting a meal.

Consider the products you use in your kitchen: dishwashing liquid, floor cleaner, surface sprays, oven cleaner, window cleaner. How do they impact your body and the environment? Have you ever considered them before, and how they might affect your health?

There are plenty of alternatives to toxic cleaners. Eco-friendly products are readily available, but you can just as easily make your own cleaning products using items you probably already have in the kitchen. I like to use lemon, vinegar, bicarbonate of soda, and eucalyptus essential oil to clean my home.

Consider how you feel when dirty dishes are left strewn all over the kitchen benches, or when there is dirt under your feet. What would your kitchen feel like if you made the time each day to keep it clean, tidy and orderly? Would this nourish you as much as the food you're preparing?

Does your kitchen feel enlivened when there are wooden bowls with limes and lemons or a pot of fresh basil? Do you feel inspired to cook when you see glass jars filled with seeds, nuts, dried fruits, legumes and beans?

Ideally, just stepping into your kitchen should ignite your creative spirit. If it doesn't, consider what it is about the space that is missing for you. Generally, the addition of plant life in the form of fresh herbs, flowers, or other greenery will make a difference.

If ever there's a place in the home to invest in slow

time, it's the kitchen. Slow food is about pleasure, and sharing, as well as being creative. Here, in the heart of the home, we are making a connection between ourselves and the world.

The Living Room

Ah, that wonderful feeling when I sink into our plum-coloured sofa, put my feet up, and grab a book to read by the woodstove. Comfort. Pleasure. That is the main purpose of the living room. Not to cook, sleep or bathe, but to relax and be with family, friends or enjoy some solitary time.

How easy it is for this room to become a dumping ground for all sorts of bits and pieces. But if this room is meant to nurture you, then in what ways can you create order and bring some structure to the space?

Baskets are a wonderful way to give things a home, whether they're children's toys, magazines, books, kindling or craft items. Oftentimes, a room loses its sense of comfort simply because we have too many things in there. As with any room in the home, paring back to essentials, and then decorating with a few items of beauty, is all it needs to make a space feel loved.

Comfort can come from throws, a basket of woolly blankets, a crystal in the window, or framed children's artwork.

Bathroom

It's the place we come to at the end of a long day: a private space, a sanctuary from the world outside. Although the kitchen is often described as the heart of the home, it could be said that the bathroom nourishes us, too. For it is here that we relieve ourselves, both physically and emotionally. We come to this hide-away to relax. In this haven, we dismantle ourselves, and put ourselves back together before entering the world again, or retiring to sleep. It's an oasis for cleansing, grooming and hygiene.

Whether we're a toddler, teenager, menstruating woman, grandparent or dad, stay-at-home mum or career woman, our vulnerable self finds a home in this space.

If the bathroom reflects our soul needs, what does yours say about you? Indeed, is it nurturing?

Use plants to clean the air, rather than chemicals to disguise unpleasant odours. Remove all toxic cleaning and body products, and replace with natural ones.

Bedroom
I love bedtime! That delicious moment when you slip onto a clean sheet, and rest your weary head on a soft pillow: Bliss. That utterly gorgeous feeling of being 'well spent' because you've fully lived your day...and by that, I don't mean you were rushed off your feet.

The human body
needs dark when asleep,
and modern lighting
hugely impacts our
hormones and happiness levels.

Rather, a well-lived day is one in which you lived it slowly enough to enjoy and appreciate every moment.

We might spend most of the time in our bedroom asleep, but that doesn't mean we should neglect it. Make sure you have a mattress that suits your body. For some reason (probably financial), we tend to use mattresses long after we should, and this isn't good for our back. Bedding is ideally made from natural fabrics. For cosy comfort, ensure your pillows and cushions feel good to you.

Does your bedroom have a high vibration? That is, do you feel good when you enter the room?

As we drift off to sleep, it's important that our body feels soothed so our mind can slip away peacefully. Keep a lavender plant by your bed, or sprinkle 100% essential oil of lavender on your pillow. It is known to soothe the weary. It's important that the air temperature in your room isn't too warm. Where possible, even in cold weather, let fresh air in through the window. If you sleep near street lighting, close the curtains. Avoid clock radios and *any* form of electric lighting while you sleep.

The human body needs dark when asleep, and modern lighting hugely impacts our hormones and happiness levels.

The sanctuary of the bedroom is best honoured by keeping it completely free of modern technology. The electro-magnetic fields emitted are not conducive to good human health and sleep patterns. These include TVs, mobile phones, clock radios, lamps, laptops, Kindle and other electronic reading devices.

Consider your bedroom as a sacred space: for sleep and lovemaking. Create a love nest, and watch your relationship change for the better.

A bedroom is an ideal place to create a small altar

Tip: apparently people with purple bedrooms have more intimacy in their relationships. Don't go off buying purple paint, though; simply add some purple touches: cushions, blankets, a picture, candles.

(assuming your bedroom is designated as sacrosanct, and not a dumping ground for laundry). Use a special cloth as the base, then add items which have meaning, such as a photo of you with your partner (if you have one), a scented rose, or bunch of lavender, some gemstones, a beeswax or plant-based candle. Allow it to become a focal point to soothe your senses. If you're not in a relationship, and would like to be in one, find an image or sculpture to symbolise what an intimate relationship means to you.

At bedtime, indulge in simple rituals to ease out of your day and prepare for sleep. This might include sipping on a mug of steamy chamomile or valerian tea. I religiously spray magnesium oil onto my skin each day. Magnesium is integral to over three hundred biochemical processes in the body. Most of us are severely deficient. Absorbing it transdermally (through

Consider your bedroom
as a sacred space:
for sleep and lovemaking.

the skin) is eight times more effective than through the digestive system. You will sleep like a baby.

Perhaps you could write by candlelight or a lamp.

Keep a gratitude journal where you write down five things from each day that you're grateful for. It will change your life.

Consider having a pamper drawer. This might include things like lip balm, an emery board, jasmine or honeysuckle oil, and inspirational reading. I love to read a book called *Heart Thoughts* by Louise L. Hay. It's a nice way to end the day. You could also try poetry or something by Kahlil Gibran.

Sleep with the window open, and allow fresh air to circulate in your bedroom. When you awaken in the morning, make your bed first thing. It's a great habit to get into, and sets the tone for the rest of the day. It makes a huge difference to how you feel when you walk into the room.

Working daily to create a serene space in your bedroom will make the world of difference to other aspects of your life. It says you care about how you rest and recuperate.

If you absolutely have to work in your bedroom (due to space restrictions), use a divider so you can't see the work station from your bed, and make sure you always switch everything off at least an hour or so before sleep.

Simplify Your Space
As we become proficient at creating our day, every detail of our lives becomes amplified, including our living space. We become conscious of everything around us. We simply must make time to declutter and simplify if we expect to feel content.

Our home is a mirror of our internal world. If you

had to pack your life into a couple of suitcases, what would you put there? What has the most meaning?

True prosperity isn't to be found in having a houseful of things. Keep what is essential, then have a few items which beautify and nourish your sacred space. Everything else is unnecessary.

It takes time, work and commitment to declutter and send things off to charity shops or for recycling, but in the end what you're doing is making far less work for yourself on a daily basis. Minimising your wardrobe will make washing and ironing less of a chore, for a start. One idea to reduce dishes is to have only one plate or bowl or cup out for each family member, and for each person to be responsible for washing and drying that dish. It'll really change your washing-up situation.

Many years ago when I worked in a Montessori school, I really appreciated that the classroom environment was clutter free and beautiful: everything had a home. The young children would take an activity off the shelf, and before they moved onto another one, they always put the first one away. Every item had a place where it belonged.

One of the reasons modern-day mums and dads (and kids) get so overwhelmed is because there is simply far too much stuff for the available living space.

Be clear: clutter is not about a shortage of storage solutions. It means we have too much stuff! When clothes don't fit easily and neatly into a wardrobe and drawers, it means you have too many. When books don't make it onto a bookshelf it means…oh wait, hang on, it means you need to buy another bookshelf (says the author with an obsession for books)! Just kidding!

Too many dishes, plates, cups, cutlery? Get rid of them. Charity shops are always wanting more things.

The Ancestor Altar

As I write, my cousin Monica is exploring our family tree and gathering lots of stories and old photos of our ancestors and ancestresses for us to enjoy. I marvel to see these people with whom I share DNA.

We are the fingertips, living out their dreams, balancing their karma, healing their wounds. Talk to your ancestors as if they were in the same room. They are. Tell them your woes. Share with them your hopes. Our ancestral heritage plays a significant role in our sense of who we are and where we've come from.

Vibrational Medicine

If there is a pattern of grief in your family line, consider the Australian Bush Flower Essence *Sturt Desert Pea*. It's invaluable for releasing such pain. Feeling homesick for family? Try Bach's *honeysuckle* flower essence.

Get Rid of the Clutter

Astrologically, the fourth house of home and ancestry, is also about the deep subconscious. It contains so much unprocessed or unaware stuff.

Clutter in our lives is an external picture of what is going on inside our minds. Do you want to think more clearly? Do you want to feel on top of your life? Then I urge you to consider all the things which fill your home (and car), and start to get rid of anything which doesn't fill you with joy. Obviously, practical things like vacuum cleaners need to stay.

If you consider your mind to be like a filing cabinet, then when there's too much stuff going in, the doors can't close properly. Chaos becomes our way of life. Likewise, our emotional life also leads to clutter. Be clear that this isn't about getting more storage solutions

Clutter in our lives
is an external picture
of what is going on
inside our minds.

for your home, but about actually releasing yourself from possessing so much stuff. Books have been one of the hardest things for me to part with because I always think someone might need a particular book one day. I am, however, learning to let go.

There are other ways to emotionally declutter, too, such as journaling or meditating. Walking, and other forms of exercise, are also powerful ways to release. Never underestimate, though, the power of a minimalist home.

When decluttering, aim to do as much as you can in one go. It needs the energy of that huge shift in order for you to be able to maintain the new space that's created. Hold each item in your hand and ask yourself if it brings you joy.

How often do we hold onto things years after they've served their purpose? How many items do we keep in storage even though we have no use for them? Let go. Free yourself. Watch your life change.

Gems & Crystals

Gems and crystals can bring healing to your home. Place a quartz crystal in each corner of a room.

Citrine is the merchant's stone. Use it to attract financial good fortune. Keep it in your purse, or by your bank statements. For health and well-being, place *celestite* in your bedroom and bathroom. Help minimise the dangerous electromagnetic radiation forces from your computer and television by placing *fluorite* around them. If your home needs calming, due to friction between family members, try *selenite*. *Haematite* may be placed near your front door to protect from any negativity which may be brought to your home.

Ways to bring life to a home

[] Open the windows every day and let fresh air and sunshine stream in.

[] Place good-sized plants in every room (and look after them).

[] Put crystals on window sills or hang them near windows to allow sunlight to cast rainbows throughout your room.

[] Sweep or vacuum each day.

[] Leave shoes at the front door, and keep the floors free of outdoor toxins.

[] Laugh a lot.

[] Play an instrument; bang a drum. Hang chimes in the window. Put on a CD.

[] If there are toxins in your home, cut an onion in half and leave it for a day or two. It will absorb them from the air. Do NOT eat the onion afterwards.

[] Invite positive friends into your living space.

Affirmations

I love my living space. It is calm, beautiful and healing.
I am safe. My home is safe.
I have the ideal living space.
I release my past. I am free from my ancestral karma.
I love my family, and my family loves me.
I am grateful for the relationship I have with my parents.
I belong.
I am free from the past.
I forgive my parents.

Aromatherapy
Sweet orange and cedar

Flower Essences
Chicory, Honeysuckle, Centaury, Red Chestnut, Chamomile, Pink Yarrow, Pomegranate, Aspen, Clematis. *Mariposa Lily* helps to calm any mother issues one may have. It is like 'mother love' in a glass bottle. Take this essence for when you feel homesick or have a deep need for mother, or for wanting a hug. It can be helpful as a 'leaving home' remedy.

Healing Modalities
Psychotherapy, inner-child work, family therapy, astrology, emotional-release work, floatation therapy, Moon water.

Meditation or Visualisation Image
In your mind, create your ideal home. Consider the material it is built from, and the location. Here, you can have any home you like, and have it anywhere in the world. Use this image to give you a sense of comfort and place. Visit this home any time you need a safe place.

Moon Water
As a child, my mother made us solarised (Sun) water. This was water which was placed in the sunlight all day, with coloured cellophane around it. Every colour had its own healing energy. We'd drink different colours depending on what we needed. For example, yellow to ease bedwetting. Blue to eliminate a headache. Red to help a shy child feel stronger.

Moon water is left outdoors during the Full Moon, and takes on the charge of the sign the Moon is in. Consider the energies of these zodiac signs, and what influences you might wish to imbibe, then task your water to take on the energy of that particular Full Moon. Make sure you cover the glass to keep insects out of it.

Aries: physical stamina, energy, drive, leadership, pioneering energy, bravery
Taurus: comfort, pleasure, money, material security
Gemini: ease of communication, local community, local travel, media, speaking, neighbours, siblings
Cancer: home, family, nurturing, emotional security, growth, ancestors
Leo: fun, play, children, creativity, joy, performance, love affairs
Virgo: nutrition, health, attention to detail, writing, perfection, editing, purification, detoxing, rituals and ceremonies
Libra: beauty, fairness, kindness, justice, relationships, marriage, romance, charm
Scorpio: honesty, depth, power, passion, mystery, sexuality, birth, death (letting go), transformation, shared resources
Sagittarius: adventure, philosophy, the search for meaning, foreign travel, university learning, seeing the bigger picture
Capricorn: practicality, earthiness, building, reputation, career, stability, fame
Aquarius: humanity, global awareness, brotherhood, revolution, eccentricity, thinking outside the box
Pisces: compassion, divinity, unity, faith, music

Heart Questions

Is my home a place where I feel safe?
Do I feel nourished within my home?
What would enhance my home?
What is my favourite room in the house, and why?
What memories do I have of my childhood home? Did I feel safe there?
What does the mother archetype mean to me?
What is the family story through the generations?

*"If the only prayer you said
in your whole life was,
'thank you', that would suffice."*
~ Meister Eckhart

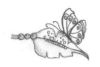

Creativity

I Create My Fun

I play, therefore I am

If we think of this area of life (the fifth house in astrology) as like a sandpit, or perhaps a sandy beach, the question to ask yourself is: how do I play?

Do you dive into the sandpit finishing your sandcastle before everyone else has even grabbed their bucket and spade? Maybe you're a loner, and would rather play by yourself. Perhaps you decorate your castle with flowers and grasses, and sea shells and colourful glasses which have been smoothed by the tides. Perhaps yours is the biggest castle of all. Maybe a sandpit is a bit too three dimensional for you, and you'd rather build your castle in cyberspace? Or the sky?

For most of my adult life, I didn't know 'how' to play. My idea of fun was reading a (non-fiction) book. But I've since learned: that is the whole point. Play and fun and pleasure are *personal*. One person's idea of fun might be to go paintballing, or car rallying across a desert, while another's is to do burlesque dancing. Another person might derive pleasure from baking cupcakes, or hanging out with a child for the afternoon doing finger painting. I love to walk in the woods, and listen to classical music. They may not sound like 'fun' activities to some people, but I derive huge amounts of pleasure from them.

We were born to create, and be creative. Many of us tend to think we don't have a creative bone in our body, but 'art' — *real* art — isn't about paints, necessarily.

Life is a canvas, and as we explore and express who we are, then we're being artists. You might express your creative side by the way you decorate your home or potter in the herb garden. It's possible your creativity is expressed by making felt dolls or photographing old cemeteries in sepia hues.

Consciously creating your day is the ultimate in creativity! You're visualising (drawing a picture in your mind) how you want your day to unfold. And then, you live it.

Creativity is what allows us to literally make the life of our dreams. It manifests when we tap into our soul energy.

Flower Essences
Desert Alchemy produces a flower essence combination called *Creative Formula*. It facilitates the process of creativity, and connects one with their inspiration by letting go of blocks. It's useful for those having trouble conceiving, as well as those who think their creative projects aren't good enough.

Nasturtium is for igniting the spark of creation. It balances yin and yang, and allows the mind and spirit to strengthen the vital life force.

GoCreate essence.

Sunflower essence. This essence allows us to shine, and is also helpful for those who need to heal their father issues. We recognise the sunflower as the brightest, biggest flower in the garden. But here's the interesting thing: we might notice those beautiful yellow petals, but what the flower is bursting to show us are its seeds: the origins of creativity. Take this essence to allow your creative spirit a place to shine.

Your Inner Artist

The Artist's Way by Julia Cameron is a wonderful book for anyone wishing to release their creativity. It's based on a 12-week self-paced course. I can't recommend it highly enough. It certainly changed the course of my life. Weekly exercises, artist dates, and daily journaling will help you root out fears and blocks about your inner artist.

Taste That Chocolate!

Did you ever read the wonderful novel by Joanne Harris called *Chocolat*? The movie is great, too. It's the story of a gypsy woman, Vianne, who ends up in a little French village and sets up a chocolate shop. During Lent! Needless to say, the town's mayor, Comte de Reynaud, gets in a tizz and tries to drive her out of town by saying her work is evil.

What I love about Vianne is that her clothes are colourful, she has an illegitimate child, and doesn't adhere to the town's religion. For these reasons and more, she doesn't fit in. However, she is friendly and optimistic, and her wonderful nature begins to attract those around her. Simply by being herself she gives others permission to be themselves.

What is interesting to me is that the archetype of this story paints a picture for us of our *inner* gypsy. Where are we that little bit wild? Or have we been so tamed that we do as we're told? What's wrong with having pleasure?

One by one, Vianne discovers the deepest needs and desires of the townsfolk, and divines the right chocolate flavour for them. She unleashes their ability to partake of pleasure.

I find this such an important story for our time. We're so busy making ends meet, and rushing from one job to another, that it's easy for everything, including eating, to be utilitarian, rather than pleasure-based.

Look around your life. Where do you actively invite pleasure to come and play?
1
2
3
4
5

In what ways can you bring even more fun into your life?
1
2
3
4
5

Affirmations

It is safe to be me.
I am a creator.
I have a great relationship with my children.
I am wonderful.
I let my light shine.
I approve of myself.
I lovingly enjoy my playful sexuality.
I am playful.
I have fun.
I am great with children.
I create fun in my day.
I create pleasure in my day.
I happily receive applause.
I have enjoyable leisure activities.
I laugh.
I play.

Colour Healing

Wear bright yellow, or place sunflowers in your home, to awaken your joyous heart. Consider making yellow solarised water (covering a glass with yellow cellophane, and leaving it in the sunshine all day), and drinking. Where can you allow more colour into your life?

1
2
3
4
5

Aromatherapy: Lime and sweet orange

Meditation or Visualisation Image

In your meditation or visualisation time, imagine yourself on a beach. Choose whether it is deserted or busy, or somewhere in-between. Gather everything necessary to build a sandcastle. Take as much time as you need to create something that feels good to you. Use this image to remind you of the importance of expressing your creativity, and to understand if you need an 'audience' to applaud your sandcastle.

Healing Modalities

Join a theatre group, a gym, any form of creativity, play therapy, get a sandpit and build a castle, body balancing, The Artist's Way. Prioritise having fun.

Heart Questions

When was the last time I really laughed?
What is fun?
When did I allow myself to play?
Did someone suppress my creativity when I was a child?
Do I actively have fun or pleasure every day?

Health & Service

I Create My Well-being

I analyse, therefore I am.

And now we come to the sixth house of astrology, which many astrologers dryly refer to as the house of day-to-day work or illness. I consider this area of the chart to be the house of *sacred ceremonies*.

For many people, health is something that little thought is given to until there's an illness. Good health isn't just about not being ill. It's far more than that. To enjoy great health means that we jump out of bed with enthusiasm and energy! It means that we don't need stimulants such as coffee or sugar, or sedatives, to get through the day or night. It means being comfortable in your skin, and glad to be alive.

Health doesn't have to be something that deteriorates with age. Yes, sure, we have years of gravity to contend with, but we can nourish and nurture our bodies in many ways so that our Winter years are just as vibrant and filled with vitality and zest for this amazing life as our early years.

There's a direct link between mind, body and soul. Indeed, when an illness manifests in the body we understand it to be the last portal, and that the 'illness' or *dis*-ease had its origins first in the mind or emotions.

Have you ever met someone who is ill and no matter what treatments or healing they have had, they just never seemed to get better? When illness begins in the emotions then a vitamin tablet or surgery is a bit like a band-aid. It doesn't heal the core wound.

We can learn a lot by understanding the astrological sixth house, for it is the house of daily rituals. In many ways, creating your day rests largely on what happens in this area of your life. For this is your foundation. When looked at in this way, it's hardly a 'dry' area of the chart, but one potentially rich with nutrients.

In the shower, I wash myself with lemon-myrtle soap, breathing in the gorgeous natural fragrance. The hot steam fills the room, and I'm energised by this stream of water flowing over my body. This is my most-favoured morning ritual. I come alive in the shower, and dream up storylines for my novels. Stepping out of the shower, I wrap a beach-sized soft towel around me.

Before getting dressed, I stand in front of the mirror. I may not have the body our culture suggests is beautiful or the 'right' shape, but regardless of that I tell my body how grateful I am for all it does.

I speak kindly to my wobbly ricotta-style belly (where I grew my two beautiful daughters), strong legs, arms, shoulders and breasts. I massage coconut oil into my face, and massage my arms and legs. It is here, in front of the mirror, that I see myself. Recently, I came across a black and white line drawing which said: *I want to be your friend.* The body replied: *I have waited my whole life to hear you say that.* I wept when I read it. We are so often at war with our bodies. It's time to change that, and make love, not war. Make friends with your body, and stop comparing yourself to other people.

My feet are bare upon the dewy grass. It's yet another one of my favourite times of the day: walking through my garden, feeling the coolness of the earth below. I am nourished as I deeply breathe in the fresh country air around me. This is slow time. This is nourishment.

My daily habits (rituals) include showering, brushing my teeth and hair, massaging magnesium oil into my skin, preparing fresh meals from scratch, listening to music, writing affirmations, daydreaming, taking vitamin and mineral supplements, and exercising.

I nurture the body's need for physical movement by doing an hour in the gym/or an aquafit class or an hour's swimming. On Saturdays, I take a class in dynamic control and stretch, to stabilise and strengthen my core muscles. Maybe I'll take a five-mile walk along the river or up some hills. I have come to learn that if I don't take care of my body it certainly won't take care of me.

Examining our daily rituals also means being aware of how we manage our time so that perhaps less is spent on things like social media, and more on doing activities which nurture us more fully. Nurturing, nourishing, cleaning, grooming, and exercising should be at the very heart of creating our day. To create a well-functioning body means investing in our selves over and over.

As a gardener, I know that when a flower doesn't bloom I need to alter the environment, not the plant! The same applies to humans. If you want to grow, thrive, flourish and blossom, then it's vital that *all* the growing conditions are in place.

Daily Rituals

Do you brush your hair (or massage your scalp, if bald) each day?

How often do you clean your hair?

Do you practise daily hygiene?

How often do you move your body? What is your favourite exercise?

How do you feel when you're touched? Do you have a sense of personal space?

Do you drink enough water?

Do you get out into the sunshine for at least half an hour?

I Am a Creator

As a child, our family grace at mealtime was not "two four six eight, bog in don't wait!" Instead, we said this:

I am a creator. By the power of my spiritualised will I consciously gather all the forces from this food and use them to create health, strength and harmony in all my bodies: physical, astral and mental. We thank Thee Father for this manifestation of Thy bounteous supply. May we use it to Thy Glory in Thy Service. Amen.

It might have been wordy, but as I look back on my childhood all I can think is: "wow". What a powerful affirmation for children to grow up with. Let me just say here: I AM so grateful for the mother I have!

Affirmations

I create my body through (type of exercise) each day/every other day.

I always work for wonderful bosses and with terrific colleagues.

I work with and for people whom I love.

I work in a great location.

I create my body.

I create excellent health.

I move easily.

I nourish myself through my daily rituals.

I am committed to getting plenty of sleep and relaxation.

I breathe deeply.

I am always improving.

I am whole.

I am healed

Every day is sacred.

I honour my daily rituals.

I prioritise my health and well-being.

Aromatherapy

Sweet orange and lime

Flower Essences

Crab Apple, Pine, Self-Heal, Zinnia, Jasmine. *Jasmine* is useful for someone who is out of touch with their soul purpose, because it helps to bring them back to the present moment. It allows one to find inspiration from where they are right now. It is great for bringing in love, and invoking optimism. Healthwise, it alleviates depression, doubts, impotence, PMT, skin issues, cramps and nervous exhaustion. It helps one to set goals, and is good for those with low self-esteem. It connects the mind, body and soul dots, and helps to activate the Universal force within the heart.

Useful things for creating positive daily rituals

[] Beeswax candles (they emit negative ions which clear toxins from indoors). Avoid petrochemical candles at all times.

[] Incense

[] 100% essential oils (cleaning, annointing & pleasure)

[] Crystals and gemstones

[] Water (drinking and bathing)

[] Fresh flowers

[] Inspirational reading

[] Gratitude journal

[] Yoga mat

[] Grass

[] Sunrise and sunset

[] Colouring-in pencils or chalk

[] Music

[] Flower or gem essences

[] A favourite mug for tea

[] Items from Nature to make a mandala

Meditation or Visualisation Image:

In your meditation or visualisation, walk into an old apothecary. Note the hand-crafted wooden shelves and drawers around the whole room. All around you are jars, vials, bottles and more, all filled with essences, oils, herbs and tinctures. You instinctively know exactly what you need to nourish yourself, and you find the remedy or healer easily. Come back to this place time and time again to make sure your health and well-being needs are met.

Healing Modalities

Flower essences, naturopathy, nutrition, homeopathy, and herbal medicine.

Heart Questions

Do I have daily rituals that enhance my journey from morning to night?

Do I value health, nutrition, well-being, hygiene, and ceremony in my life?

Do I consistently listen to my body's messages?

In what ways do I align my body, mind and soul?

What rituals can I incorporate in my daily life?

Am I conscious of my daily habits? How can I make them into mindful rituals?

Secrets of a Happy Life

Studies of cultures where people have happy, long lives, show they all have the following in common:

Daily exercise
Relaxation
Strong sense of community
Spirituality of some description
Enjoyable social life
Strong family bonds

A loving marriage is about mutual support and empowerment, and never about suppression.

Partnerships

I Create Loving Relationships

I balance, therefore I am

One of the things I really love about relationships is that they are ever-renewing. On any given day, we can start again, and bring something new and wholesome to the interaction. The other person is always our mirror. If we don't like what we see, there's no point throwing a hairbrush at the mirror. We have to change our view of it, and sometimes that means walking away from a relationship that doesn't respond to love, kindness, fairness and honesty. It is never a failure to end a relationship.

Any relationship we have in life is only as good and functional as our degree of self-love. The way people treat us is in direct proportion to the way we treat ourselves. When we have good strong boundaries, then

131

we tend to move through life in a way that only brings us loving and healthy relationships. When people come along who are toxic, we either don't attract them into our orbit (for long, or at all) or we move away. It's that simple. *Like attracts like.*

You might have been in an abusive relationship and are saying "hang on a minute, but I didn't abuse him!" No, but you may have abused yourself. You stayed there long enough that he was able to identify your core wound and pick at it. When you heal a wound like that, you simply can't attract abusers. There isn't the magnetism or matching vibrational frequency.

In the same way, a little girl might spend years being sexually abused, powerless to stop the perpetrators. Each time she's assaulted, the hole in her aura becomes bigger, and acts like a neon light to anyone of the paedophile disposition. She may spend her adult years attracting the same violation, or she may find a way to heal herself, thereby preventing any future abuse.

Gratitude
Give thanks for the relationships in your life. All of them. If there are ones that have outdone their time, give thanks, and let them go.

I begin my day by thanking the Universe for my husband beside me. I give thanks for our beautiful marriage, and the joy and love he brings me.

A couple of times now, when I've been thanking my husband for his presence in my life or saying "I love you, Paul" (in my *mind*, not out loud) he has woken up with a start, and asked "What did you say?" Cute!

I give thanks for all the important relationships in my life.

Allow yourself to feel all the blessings your loved

ones bring you, and name those blessings. Truly give thanks.

Being grateful is like putting money in the bank…it just keeps building up, and it attracts interest.

Relationships act like a mathematical equation where if one side of it is changed, the other side has to change. If we don't like the way a relationship is then rather than blaming the other, we look at our own behaviour and either change it or speak up (in a loving way).

Humans are creatures of habit, and if you've spent years putting your partner down or letting yourself be spoken to in a degrading way, then you need to understand that it takes two to create a healthy relationship. Change the music, and find a way to learn new steps.

When one person starts to empower themselves, the other can often find themselves stumbling and wondering what alien landscape they've walked into. If you find yourself being thwarted in your attempts to live authentically, then perhaps it's time to look more closely at what exactly that relationship brings to you.

People often suppress huge parts of themselves in an attempt to 'save' a marriage. Any marriage worth saving doesn't involve self-sacrifice. A loving marriage is about mutual support and empowerment, and never about suppression.

When you see your intimate other first thing in the morning, what is your natural response? What are the first words you speak? Do you make time to touch, to kiss, and to whisper your love?

When you spend time together (minus the children), is it free of distractions, such as TV, Facebook, mobile phones? Are you truly being present with each other?

It is often said, in our culture, that you really have to

work at marriage; that it's hard and difficult. I believe this is akin to saying that giving birth is hard and painful. Wisdom lives within us, and just as the truth is that birth can be easy, ecstatic, beautiful, painless and empowering, so too can marriage. Why does one couple struggle to coexist while another couple thrives? Is it a matter of what we've had modelled to us, or what we *believe* to be true about relationships? The core fear of separation is abandonment. It taps into our primal terror of mother leaving us. When we can acknowledge this, and work with the truth of these fears, then we stop laying the blame at the feet of our partner.

The key to a healthy and vibrant marriage lies with self-awareness. The more we can understand our own drivers and fault lines, the more we're able to meet our partner as a whole being rather than as a needy toddler who never got enough love from their parents.

Dysfunctional marriage stems from unmet childhood needs from one or both people. Rarely does it happen that a healthy, whole, integrated person ends up with someone of the opposite nature who is completely dysfunctional. We instinctively choose partners who will help us *heal old wounds*. The key to understanding our pain, though, is that it can damn well hurt when someone picks at the scab. No one wants to look inside and see what the discomfort is all about. It's far better to put on a band-aid and tell the other person to stop picking on you!

To blame our partner for our marital troubles is to miss the whole picture. While it is true that not all relationships are meant to last a lifetime, and that there are situations where it is healthier for all concerned to part ways, let's look at how to help a current relationship flourish.

*The key to a
healthy and vibrant marriage
lies with self-awareness.*

What does intimacy mean? We may talk about it meaning that we're close to a person, emotionally, sexually, intellectually, physically or spiritually. But let's break the word down: *in to me see*. Again, we come back to the idea that by looking within our self we can make great discoveries. The more we know who we are, the stronger we are in any relationship (with a life partner, business partner, best friend, child, enemy, authority figure, mentor/counsellor).

Many people believe the key to a good marriage is having lots of sex. While there's no doubt that the 'right kinda loving' can make for a pleasurable life (and lots of oxytocin helps us feel loved), lovemaking isn't just about penetration and what we do between the sheets. Lovemaking is something which can (and should) take place throughout the day, every day. It happens when our hearts connect. We woo our partner when we make eye contact and smile open-heartedly. We make love when we place our hand on their shoulder or make them a cup of tea without having to ask. We're 'made love to' when our partner can read our emotional barometer

The core fear of separation
is abandonment.
It taps into our primal terror
of mother leaving us.

just by looking at us. Lovemaking is shared through kind words, by listening fully, and not with one eye on the sports news or while reading the paper.

Listening means being 100% attentive, and recognising that most of our communication comes, in fact, through body language, rather than our spoken words.

What is the difference between lovemaking and rape? You might think the answer is obvious: one is gentle and one is violent. One is based on mutual consent, and the other is based on someone violating the other. If we consider that rape is 'being taken against our will', and usually done violently and with complete lack of respect, then the truth is that many people are in marriages where emotional and mental rape are frequent occurrences. When we blame or shame our partner, when we yell at them (for whatever reason) because we're trying to lay the fault on their doorstep, instead of owning our feelings about how we see the situation: when we only speak in sarcastic tones...*these are all abusive ways to behave.* If this is our normal mode of relating to our partner, then they'll never be able to open up to us (literally or metaphorically) and be truly intimate. If someone raped you, you wouldn't trust that they could be kind and gentle with you another time, so why would we expect any differently in an emotional or mental comparison? To open ourselves to another human being in the most intimate of ways (not just physically), we need to feel safe, secure, valued and loved. If we don't have this, we close down. And we keep closing down until there's nothing of our true selves available for the other person to relate to.

We learn basic trust from our mother. Was she there for us? Did she meet our needs? Did she change our nappy early enough? Did she provide us with food before hunger caused pain in our tiny belly? *These are the foundation stories of trust.* Did mother enjoy holding us against her bosom? We learnt about love in the arms of our mother, and about relationships from our parents (whether or not they were together during our childhood).

When we feel we can't trust our partner, it is because at the deepest level we don't trust ourselves to have our needs met. We are waiting, reliant, on another to meet our needs. We might blame our partner for having an affair and that's our reason not to trust, but if we do some soul-searching we might find a place within ourselves that didn't trust them long before the alleged crime took place. Please note, I'm not suggesting for a minute that you caused your partner to have an affair, but that the resonance within you perhaps precipitated it.

The analogy of the onion comes in quite well here. We have layers and layers of pain that have built up. It is a natural response to want to 'cover up' and protect ourselves from pain: rejection, abandonment, neglect, isolation. Humans instinctively seek pleasure, and not pain; so if pain comes in the course of day-to-day living, then we'll keep adding those onion layers to hide away our wounded heart. When one or each of you is bound in countless layers, it is very hard to 'see' the real person, and to own your authenticity. It's too deeply buried. To get to the heart of the onion means being prepared to be vulnerable and shed the layers.

A common complaint in new parents is the lack of libido which can accompany breastfeeding. At one level, this is a natural phase for the body. The time to nurture a young one should be a sacrosanct space. Men who feel jealous of the new mother-child bond would do well to investigate their mothering wounds and recognise that their inner-boy's needs were not met. If they had been, he'd be able to stand strongly and proudly as protector of the space in which he has helped create. If this complete lack of interest in lovemaking continues, it's worth checking your nutritional status, as you could be deficient in magnesium (treat it transdermally) and zinc (eat a handful of pumpkin seeds each day).

A loving couple will be able to express their sexuality in various ways, without putting pressure on the other to 'perform'. A person who receives ample touch during the day (including long hugs) will feel nurtured and loved. Sexuality is the same energy as that of creativity. If, for whatever reason, you're unable to have sex with your partner, consider if you're allowing room in your life to express yourself in other ways.

As mentioned, the vast majority of human communication takes place through body language. Spend some time observing yourself. What does your face say? What do your arms say? Is your posture relaxed, and inviting? Do you smile or scowl? Are your arms crossed in defence? Are you in warrior mode all the time? Do you turn your back on your partner when they speak? Do you even bother making eye contact? We 'speak' in a thousand ways every day. Make every gesture and word be of love, gratitude and devotion, and watch your relationships flourish!

Humour can oil the wheels of any relationship. It can be effective in defusing tense situations, and can raise the spirits when life is challenging and there's no obvious way around whatever the difficulty is. Not everyone is a humorist, but most of us appreciate humour. As long as the people sharing the joke are on a similar wavelength, and the fun is well intentioned and not at somebody's expense, then the ensuing laughter can lighten life considerably. If there's awareness in a relationship, then the humorist will generally manage to hit the spot with what they say (or do), and when they say it.

Without respect, it is impossible to maintain a loving relationship. This is often the reason a marriage breaks down. When we lose reverence for our partner, then our desire to nourish and nurture the relationship wanes, and eventually everything that was once special and important erodes before our eyes. And perhaps this is where the idea of marriage being 'hard work' comes into play. It can be hard to respect a partner who doesn't contribute to the relationship emotionally, intellectually or physically. If we feel that our loved one is more interested in a night at the pub with mates, or spending every weekend doing something we don't like, then we pull apart. We don't feel valued. We wrap another layer of the onion around ourselves. He, in turn, loses sight of the person he fell in love with.

Although we come together as individuals, a relationship is a composite of the two energies, and is an 'entity' in its own right. Therefore, a *relationship* needs to be seen and nurtured as much as the person to whom we're relating.

At the heart of respect lies common courtesy, something which seems uncommon in our modern culture. Kindness heals every relationship, even if we choose to move our separate ways.

For any relationship to be successful, it requires balancing personal needs with the needs of a couple, and the needs of a family. Within balance comes the art of compromise. It's impossible to have a happy relationship without it. And herein lies the irony: in order to flourish in the dance of marriage, it means knowing which parts of our self to let go of in order to become one. There is an element of compromise that is called for, but this should never be confused with surrender or martyrdom. For example, one half of the partnership is an extrovert and wants to spend every weekend out and about visiting people, but the other person doesn't. She wants to stay home. That's her idea of a fun weekend. A balance might look like this: every second weekend is spent honouring the other's needs. Alternatively, they agree that he can go out (with or without the children) and she can stay home. It would be wholly unbalanced if she were expected to go out every weekend.

It is said that opposites attract. To a certain extent this might be true, but this isn't necessarily sustainable over the long term. What truly attracts us to another person is when they 'see' us as we are without trying to change us to fit their needs and desires.

Balance in a relationship has to exist, even though the axis of that may shift from time to time. It doesn't have to be 50/50, but if the marriage is to work then an equal balance at some level must exist in what is essentially a symbiotic relationship.

Own your feelings. No one else can make you mad, sad, angry, happy, or grateful. You choose those feelings in response to a thought. Taking responsibility for your emotions means that you will move away from blaming your partner.

By looking within, you can come to understand what it is within you that needs to be healed. Stay present when your partner is experiencing their pain, but don't rescue them. Listen, care, empathise, but don't rescue.

Self-knowledge is at the heart of a thriving relationship. In my case, Paul and I were attracted to each other straight away, and because we were both interested in personal growth/spiritual development, we already had some insights into ourselves. We found understanding ourselves and each other in this way to be helpful. Primarily we used the Enneagram of Personality Types, but as I developed my passion for psychological astrology this helped me improve and refine my knowledge and understanding of mine and my husband's needs (and our children's).

Ideally, both partners show generosity of spirit linked with self-awareness and awareness of others. This includes self-knowledge, self-respect and self-love.

Nurturing and loving oneself, when done with awareness, becomes a foundation for loving those around us. If there's some level of self-awareness at the beginning of a relationship, the couple will have more of a chance of knowing whether they should even be together at all. It also gives them a better chance of evolving together, which is critical in preserving a relationship.

What are we teaching our children? Whether you are in a loving marriage or relationship, or widowed, or in the process of separating, or have long been apart from your child's other parent, you are *always* modelling to your children what marriage means, and how it can enhance or destroy a person's life. Some people, who haven't had a strong and authentic model of a loving marriage, learn to model their own on the Divine Union: a blend of the masculine and feminine; protector and nurturer; giver and receiver. People who stay in unhappy marriages 'for the sake of the children' are missing something very important: they're teaching children that it is better to be unhappy than to be authentic, and that marriage is, essentially, a miserable prison. The truth is that a conscious marriage can be one of the most liberating relationships to be in, in which both people grow, thrive and flourish. Focus on what is good in your partner, rather than being a nit-picker. Your job is to love, not to change the other.

In each and every one of us, there exists a place deep within the heart where we haven't been hurt. If we make a practice of accessing this place of stillness, then we can transform an average or unhappy relationship. The choice and the power is always with us. The heart chakra is our centre. In the chakra colour chart, it is green: the colour of balance. By closing your eyes, and imagining yourself centred into this part of your being, you can find all the answers you need to nurture your relationship (yes, even if you're divorced).

Learning to love yourself is vital if you expect to allow others into your heart space. Avoid taking your partner for granted. Relationships (even those 'bound' in law or in the eyes of God) are a *choice*. No one has to stay there. Make a conscious choice, every single day, to be 100% there for your partner, and just as importantly for yourself.

Forgiveness brings freedom, and allows us to let go of the past. There are many ways to learn the art of letting go, releasing and moving on. You could, for instance, learn *Ho'oponopono*, an ancient Hawaiian practice of reconciliation and forgiveness.

Although the decision to break up the living arrangements of a family is not something to be taken lightly, it can be done amicably and with love, care and reverence for all concerned. Try to avoid being a parent who uses the children to avenge the pain you

143

feel at your former partner. They're not your weapons. They are living beings who have a right to love both parents, and be loved by them. Let all your choices be for the highest good of all concerned. Speak the highest image of your former partner that you can so that your children can see that you are a magnanimous human being.

Separation can be a vulnerable and difficult time for all concerned. My dear friend, the late Jeannine Parvati Baker, wrote movingly about the biological story inherent within us as the genetic legacy of love: *each child has both parents in every cell of their body*. Despite the biological truth that the mother provides more genetic material, we are made of almost equal proportions of our parents' DNA. What does this mean? When you talk about the child's other parent, the child hears the message of who they are on the deepest cellular level. Jeannine described it beautifully when she said, "There are ears within the ten-billion cells of my children that take the stories in deeply. Not only in my children dwell the DNA of their father, but in my brainstem and bloodstream as well".

When a woman conceives, the father's genetic material migrates into her. If the pregnancy is viable, and the mother gives birth, there's a huge migration of the father's DNA into her body. Therefore, for each child that a woman has with a man, the more of his genetics are lodged within her.

Talk about your child's father (or mother) as if they were right there with you, witnessing everything you say. Be loving, forgiving, honest, open and grateful.

If you find it hard to consider anything positive about your ex-partner, simply look into the face of your child (children), and be <u>grateful</u> that your relationship

*"When parents fight,
it's the equivalent of war, to the child."*
~ Anaïs Nin

produced such a beautiful being. Gratitude is as powerful a force as love, and it can transform lives.

Very few people stay conscious on their journey through separation and divorce; and yet, if they were to retain the keys of intimacy: communication, respect and trust, they'd find the journey of parting ways to be empowering, supportive and loving for all concerned.

As a celebrant, I offer divorce ceremonies. Most people laugh at the irony of a marriage celebrant doing that, but it can be a beautiful, healing and sacred time for both people. It allows them to honour and value everything that was good in their time together, and to part ways with love, honesty and gratitude. The ceremony also offers them the chance to burn away all that hadn't been positive in their union, and release it with gratitude and love. There are times in life to stay together, and there are times in life when we need to move on. Admittedly, some relationships are easier than others. Even in the best of relationships, the partner often provides the perfect 'hook' for our wounds.

Without trust, there is no point to a relationship. Trust is our hope, conviction, confidence and expectation that the marriage has meaning, value, love and respect. When we don't trust our partner, it is always worth looking within and asking what it is about ourselves that we don't trust. What are we withholding? What are we denying? Where are we withholding our authenticity? If we can genuinely look inside and see that we're not contributing to the healthy well-being of the relationship, then it may be time to walk away or make huge steps towards personal transformation. Where do we go from there? Back to the beginning. We learn about who we are, and what we attract. We learn about communication in all its forms. We learn about where we give our power away, and where we hold it back. First and foremost, we forgive our parents for *anything* which may have seeded a belief that we weren't worthy, or that relationships weren't happy places to be. We learn about love, reverence, balance and respect. When we can do all of these things for ourselves, then we will attract a partner worthy of our being. We all deserve to love and be loved. It is our birthright.

There's a backpack we wear when we enter a relationship, whether it be platonic or sexual. In that small piece of luggage are the stories and wounds from childhood and ancestrally. The thing about the backpack is that we're so used to carrying it around, that it is as if it's not even an attachment, but glued to us. Those wounds and stories become patterns in our subconscious which then become belief systems. Our 'reality', then, is based on a lifetime of storytelling, both personal, familial and cultural.

We don't see the world as it is, or the 'other' as they are, but as we are. How we interact in relationship is

*The truth is that
a conscious marriage
can be one of the most
liberating relationships to be in,
in which both people grow,
thrive and flourish.*

like trying to discover who we are by looking into the other person as if they're a mirror.

When I was younger, I believed 'all men are bastards'. This was my mantra. I really don't know where I got such a thought from, as my dad certainly wasn't one, but he did impact me hugely by his absence. He worked overseas throughout my childhood. When my mother discovered she was pregnant with me, he was already back overseas. She told him of my existence in a letter. Before I was even born, I was picking up the idea, on a cellular level, that 'men aren't available'.

I have countless childhood memories of waving my father off at the airport, and sobbing my heart out. Abandonment wounds run deep.

Inevitably I created relationships with men who were unavailable in one form or another: workaholics, married to someone else, geographically distant, and emotionally absent.

I'll always be grateful to a boss of mine, as I mentioned earlier, that I worked with in the personal-growth field, who pointed out to me one day that I had to change my beliefs about men if I wanted to change my experiences of them. Could he be right? I wondered.

It was through working with him, and discovering

that there were good men in the world, that I allowed myself to believe it was a possibility that I'd meet a man who was kind, loving and available. As I've shared, within weeks, Paul walked into my life. It was a fundamental change in my thinking which allowed me to create a portal into my new reality.

Relationships of all sorts are a reflection of where we are in life. They are where we project the parts of us we disown. We do not have to be a victim of our previous experiences. The power to change is within us.

In astrology, we look to the seventh house of a person's natal chart to see what they 'project' onto their significant other (or business partner/counsellor). In my case, it's humour. I love to laugh, and in Paul I have found someone who has me laughing all day long. I don't feel humour comes naturally to me, and I look in the mirror of relationship to live out this disowned part of me. So there is a truth to the saying that opposites attract.

One of the biggest difficulties in relationships comes about because of our wounding. It is only when we've broken the umbilical cord with our parents, and have healed (or come to terms with) our childhood pain and patterns, that we can enter relationships as an adult: whole.

It's an interesting fact that we're attracted to people who have a similar smell to us. It's a biological certainty. But what happens when we wear high-strength deodorants and antiperspirants or go on the contraceptive pill (which changes our hormonal balance, and sense of smell)? How do we know we're attracting the right person for us? It's been found that women's hormones change dramatically when taking chemical/synthetic hormones, and that the man they might be attracted to while on contraception could change when they come off it, for example, to create children. Why aren't we taught this in school?

When we look at our stories, our wounds, and our patterning, we must take into account one of the cultural stories, which is that: a human shouldn't smell human. We shouldn't smell of sexual arousal, sweat, breast milk, and so on. Yet, smell is an important human sense! When we deny it, then something fundamental is missing from our relationships.

Regardless of our spiritual or religious beliefs, there exists within each of us a memory of the place we came from before we took on life in a physical body. Some people spend their lives in devotion to something Greater than themselves: a yearning for something more. For most people, however, there is a search for something that will remind us of 'home'. One of the biggest cultural stories is one indoctrinated into little girls from a young age: Prince Charming (aka Mr Right). We are conditioned to believe there is one man (or woman) out there, somewhere, waiting for us. The truth is that there are probably *dozens* of really suitable 'soulmates' for us on this planet. If we believe that there can only possibly be one 'right' person for us, we may miss out on potential beautiful relationships.

Again, our cultural conditioning sets us up to believe that marriage is the beginning of a daydreamy-honeymoon life where we'll gaze into each other's eyes forever. No wonder people divorce! Marriage includes the harsh reality of things like washing dirty nappies, bills, snoring, dirty socks, illness, demanding children, earning an income, sleep deprivation, hormonal fluctuations, and sharing time with friends. One of the biggest contributors to gulfs in a relationship is when a lover becomes a mother. No longer is she getting dressed up to go on hot dates with her man. He's unlikely to want to woo a woman with bags under her eyes, who no longer feels like sex, and has breast-milk-soaked pyjamas. What do we do?

The key is for each of us to 'own' whatever it is we're looking for in the other. So, if a man is looking for a beautiful, feminine woman, and he's instead facing an exhausted, harried mum trying to feed three children breakfast, he could look for the feminine within himself. The more he can do this, the less chance there is of him belittling his wife or being frustrated by her. Equally, a woman who was first attracted to that strong man and now finds he's not nearly as much of a hero as she first thought, can find ways to access her inner warrior. Perhaps she could take up weight-resistance training or join a karate class? When we own our inner feminine and masculine, we liberate our partner enormously.

When my younger daughter was sixteen, she had homework for philosophy class which asked: who are you? How often do we label ourselves by our roles? Mother, wife, friend, writer (fill in job title)…

Until we know who we are, then we're going to project a lot of what we *don't know about ourselves* onto our partner. It is the day when you can look in the mirror and see yourself and say "I know who I am", that everything changes. We realise we don't need anyone else in our life to 'fulfil' us, but we consciously choose our relationships based on preference rather than subconscious patterns. We come together not out of infantile needs, but adult consciousness.

We stop using relationships as therapy to heal the wounds of childhood, and instead enjoy them because our own sun is shining brightly. Loving your own company is a good indicator of how you are likely to fare in relationships. It doesn't mean you don't like being with other people, but that you take pleasure in the time you spend with yourself. When we love to 'hang out' with ourselves, then we become the sort of person other people enjoy being with too.

A consequence of growing and changing is that some relationships in our life may fall by the wayside. This may seem tragic or traumatic at the time, but it is a sign that you are integrating and owning your projections. Ironically, it is a good thing!

A healthy relationship is one where the individuals are focused on intimacy (*in to me see*), and are open to change. It doesn't involve a parent-child symbiosis, but is of one adult relating to another adult.

Communication is honest, open, passionate and assertive. Each person is capable of being independent, and the relationship is always based on trust. The roles aren't static, but always growing, evolving and changing. Honesty is the highest form of intimacy.

Attracting Your Soulmate

Devote your energy to becoming the best version of yourself that you can be. Be someone that another would enjoy hanging out with. Ignore the expression: misery loves company. I can assure you, misery is *not* an attraction, and the right sort of company will not enjoy it.

Discover the joy and zest for life within you, and let that light shine brightly.

Invest time, love, money and happiness into the relationship you have with yourself.

Treat others how you would wish to be treated.

When you have a healthy level of self-awareness,

respect and love, you will start vibrating in such a way that similar types of people will be drawn into your world.

Write a list of everything that you desire in a relationship (keep it positive, always focusing on what you want rather than what you don't want).

Rewrite your list every day, and make sure that you write it in order of priority. Some days, your desires will change order. That's okay, just remember to write each day. You will become clearer about what is important to you, hence the shifting order.

Affirmations
I am loving and loveable.
I create beautiful relationships in every area of my life.
I am conscious in all my interactions.
My relationships are a mirror, and I love what I see.
I enjoy harmonious relationships.
I attract loving people into my world.
I enjoy committed relationships filled with love and joy.
I live in balance and harmony.

Aromatherapy
Pink grapefruit and lemon

Flower Essences
Red Clover, Calendula, Eucalyptus, Holly, Agrimony, Sweet Pea. *Holly* is a great essence for those who are jealous or experience envy in relationships.

If you felt rejected in childhood, *Evening Primrose* flower essence will help to deal with those feelings of abandonment so you don't recreate them in adult relationships.

If you find yourself habitually arguing with your

partner, try *Calendula* flower essence.

If you have recently come to the end of a relationship, consider the flower essence *Bleeding Heart* to help you through your pain.

Meditation or Visualisation Image
In your meditation or visualisation, witness an elderly couple on either side of a see-saw, finding balance. They're laughing about the wonderful life they've had together, and what a joy it was to have found each other. Feel their love, and let it find a place in your heart where you know that we all have a soulmate who sees us only through the eyes of love.

Healing Modalities
Acupuncture, biofeedback, co-counselling, relationships counselling, body balance.

Heart Questions
What has been my experience of intimate relationships?
Is there a recurring theme to my relationships?
Do I feel safe to open up and share my true self?
Do I feel worthy of an intimate other?
Would I like to attract a soulmate?
How might a soulmate change my life?
What was my parents' relationship like? What have I learnt about relating from them?

Honesty is the highest form of intimacy.

Transformation

I Create Intimacy

I desire, therefore I am

Astrologers of old called the eighth house the House of Death. Well wouldn't that scare the crap out of you if you had planets there? As a modern astrologer (and hopefully more enlightened when it comes to the understanding of this), I call it the *House of Transformation*.

I don't believe that someone with an accented eighth house is necessarily going to experience more physical deaths in their lifetime than other people, however they will learn about dying. By this, I mean, they'll understand about surrender, and 'dying' unto another person or transformative experience.

This area of life is about shared resources, so includes things like money we receive without having to work for it (such as inheritances or a partner's income), debts, sexuality. Astrologically, I look to this part of the chart to see how my client experiences 'sharing'. One way of understanding this is to consider what happens when we have an orgasm. Most people would think it is simply physical, and is something the other person *causes* you to experience. An orgasm simply can't happen in the physical body without our brain giving the body permission. In other words, we have to 'let go' and surrender in order to experience those rather delicious fireworks. Our partner, skilled or otherwise, may be engaging with us sexually, but it is through our own 'death', that is, a letting go of control, that we come to enjoy the climax our Creator so wisely blessed us with receiving.

I use orgasm as an example of 'death', because the same idea applies to other aspects of true intimacy. The more open, honest and true we are with ourselves, then the more fluently we experience our intimate actions with other people, especially in relation to shared resources.

Astrologically, we include birth in this house. You might wonder what birth, death, other people's money and sex could all have in common to be lumped into one house. I'd like to share a personal story.

Throughout childhood, from an early age, I was sexually abused by various men: a kindergarten teacher, an uncle, neighbourhood men, a worker on our farm. Wounds like that shape you. They alter your sense of self, and can cause one to have unstable or malleable boundaries. This 'pattern' continued until my early adult years when a male employer sexually harassed me in the workplace. Funny how in childhood it's called abuse, but in adulthood we simply call it 'harassment' as if it's a mere inconvenience rather than a violation.

Long story short: I found my voice and spoke up. I was working in a hospital laboratory at the time, and as it turned out there were no laws in place to protect women in Queensland hospitals from this sort of behaviour. By speaking up, I can guarantee you that there is now legal protection! This was the beginning of me learning to stand up for myself, and to recognise where I ended and another person started.

When I gave birth to my older daughter, several years later, I birthed her peacefully by candlelight in the privacy of my bedroom, and the comfort of a warm birthing pool. A woman is never more open—physically or psychologically—than when she opens her legs to give birth. If ever there's a time to see your sexuality manifest, it's in the birthing process. I surrendered fully to my baby emerging from me, and she entered this world easily and peacefully. The pool gave me a physical boundary so I could open up (on every level), and know I was not going to be violated. The sexual healing that occurred on that Autumn night in New Zealand was unlike anything I've ever experienced. This is what transformation looks like. It's when we take one thing and it is turned to gold through alchemy. Of course, you don't have to have such drastic scenarios to witness transformation in your life.

This area of life is also around 'power games'. This may manifest in bullying, for example, or other ways people try to control us. If this area of life sounds all gloom and doom, please know that it doesn't have to be like that at all. It's a deep house, that's for sure, but the rewards of crossing to the other side are enormous. It can be deeply healing.

The Green Grass

The energy of this house may amplify our inherent potential for jealousy. It happens when we believe someone has something we want (and perhaps, may never have). From where we stand, the grass is greener on their side of the fence. We want to kick their damn white picket fence down and demand to know why they have the perfect life. How unfair!

The grass is greener where we water it. If you keep focusing on what someone else has, the grass beneath your feet will wither and die. *Put your attention on what you have*. Be grateful for what and whom you already have in your life. Focusing on lack only creates more lack. There's a reason why that old Bible warns against coveting your neighbour's wife. It's not to make you feel guilty but to tell you to focus on your own garden, chappy.

By all means be inspired by another person's life, but refrain from jealousy, as the only person to be hurt is yourself. It's also an unspoken message to the Universe that you don't believe you're worthy of creating the life of your dreams.

Gratitude During Grief

When my father was killed in a car accident four years ago, I experienced a grief both raw and pummelling. It threw my world upside down. Ours hadn't been the easiest relationship, because of the 'abandonment issues' about him being an absent father due to him working overseas for months at a time. One of the things that strikes me about the period after his death, in particular, was the path of spiritual grace that I walked. He was killed in Australia, and I was living in the UK. The angels arranged for me to buy a long-haul flight at short notice. I was so grateful that my passport was up to date. I knew that I didn't need to physically be there, and that I could have had my own ritual and farewell ceremony here, but something strong pulled at me to fly to my homeland. This was the first time that all of us eight children were ever together at the same time. It was an amazing experience, despite the grief. I was so grateful for this time.

To stand at 7.30am and feel good ol' Queensland sunshine bringing warmth to my body filled me with immense gratitude. I've really missed proper hot sunshine while living in England.

I was grateful that my younger sister, Ramona, created a ceremony which truly reflected Dad's passions and joys. It really made my heart sing to see how well she had personalised everything.

What I was not expecting, when I travelled across the globe, was that I would see my father's body. It hadn't even occurred to me, but when my sister said the casket was open, and asked if I wanted to see him, I knew straight away that the answer was yes.

That feeling I had, as I stood by his side, is still as strong today. I held his hand, and said "Thank you so much for everything, Dad. Thank you for working so hard for all those years so we could have a beautiful home, and the amazing childhood that we had on the land. Thank you."

Dad's hands were just as I'd remembered them: calloused. There were working man's hands. In death, I was able to speak to my father in ways I never had in life.

I am so grateful that I chose him for my father, for he provided me with many invaluable lessons, and in many ways was a great role model. I'm grateful that his DNA is in my body, and that his sense of ambition, perseverance, and self-belief are encoded into my cells. Thank you, Dad.

A friend said to me, a couple of years later, how much my father's death had changed me. I wasn't sure what she meant, but I can really see it now. My father was one of the hardest-working people I've ever met. He was a pioneer, visionary, a leader, and left a real legacy of creativity and business acumen. But as I stood by his body that sunny day, it hit me hard in the chest: *you can't take it with you when you go.* Of course, this is something I always knew intellectually. No matter how much money you earn, or what you own, the only thing that you take with you when you leave this Earth is the love of friends and family. Somehow, though, I really felt what this meant. I thought of everything my father had achieved, and how that seemed, in some ways, irrelevant. What was it all for, I wondered. My attitude to life has changed enormously since that time. I feel less stressed about achieving things, and recognise that the true legacy of what I leave behind isn't about my work, but about the time I spend with people I love. I am grateful for this life lesson.

Dealing with the Dark Clouds of Depression
It's not unusual for a person with planets in the eighth house to experience depression. Of course, there may be biological reasons for this just as there may be life events which have triggered the experience. The brain needs feeding. This obviously begins from the moment of conception, and how our mother's experience of pregnancy shapes our growing self. After we're born, there is only one food suitable for the optimal development of the infant brain: *human breast milk,*

160

ideally from the mother. The brain needs this for a minimum of two and half years, and ideally up to the age when the first milk teeth come out.

If you or someone you know experiences depression, consider natural ways to feed your brain that don't involve drugs. For example, magnesium is the number -one nutrient in brain health. It works in the same way as lithium does for those with bipolar disorder, but without it being a drug. Consider including 3-4 dessertspoons of organic virgin coconut oil in your daily diet. These brain foods nourish and allow healing.

If your depression is due to inadequate nourishment (physical or psychological) in infancy, you need to find ways to build new neural pathways by inviting conscious pleasure into your daily life. No one else can do this for you. Empower yourself by taking baby steps each day towards wholeness. It is a statement of truth that we don't see the world as it is, but as we are. If the world is looking bleak, then it is time to go inwards and discover what is lurking in the depths. Monsters won't survive if they're doused in love, kindness and awareness.

Aromatherapy
Tangerine and black spruce

Flower Essences
Holly, Rock Rose, Chicory, Honeysuckle, Sweet Chestnut. To help someone prepare for death, offer them *Angel's Trumpet* flower essence.

If the dying person needs support on a spiritual level, offer *Angelica. Borage* (starflower) can help the loved ones of the dying/deceased to find courage.

161

When questioning our own mortality, *Chrysanthemum* helps us get in touch with our Higher Self.

Affirmations
I am grateful that I always have the money to pay my bills.
I am thankful for the compliments I receive.
I am happy that other people experience good luck, and I know there is plenty for me, too.
I enjoy a healthy approach to sex.
I own my beliefs.
I am powerful, and empowered.
I release old patterns.
I give birth easily.
I surrender, and receive.
I am able to safely share.
There is plenty for everyone in this world, including me.

Meditation or Visualisation Image
In your meditation or visualisation, stand at the edge of a well. You lower a bucket tied to a rope. You wonder if you'll ever get to the life-saving water, but then you feel the bucket make contact. It's so far below. You can't see it, you can only *feel* it. Slowly, you bring the water back up and drink from the bucket, all the while knowing that you need to keep half of it for the person standing near you.

Healing Modalities
Astrology, sex therapy, depth psychology, colonic irrigation, bereavement counselling, firewalking, soul-retrieval therapy

Heart Questions

Do I need to forgive someone?
Do I need to forgive myself?
Am I at ease, sexually?
How do I feel about my sexual organs?
What is my experience of menarche/menstruation/
menopause/childbirth?
How do I feel about sharing bank accounts with my partner?
Do I feel that a parent should leave an inheritance for their
child?
Have I experienced deep grief in my life?
What was my first experience of death?
What are my beliefs about death and an afterlife?

"If we can accept that we are the sum total
of all past thoughts, emotions, words,
deeds and actions, and that our present lives and choices
are coloured or shaded by this memory bank of the past,
then we begin to see how a process
of correcting or setting aright can change our lives,
our families and our society."

~ Morrnah Nalamaku Simeona

The Twelve Principles of Attitudinal Healing

1. The essence of our being is love
2. Health is inner peace. Healing is letting go of fear
3. Giving and receiving are the same
4. We can let go of the past and of the future
5. Now is the only time there is, and each instant is for giving
6. We can learn to love ourselves and others by forgiving rather than judging
7. We can become love-finders rather than fault-finders
8. We can choose and direct ourselves to be peaceful inside regardless of what is happening outside
9. We are students and teachers to each other
10. We can focus on the whole of life rather than the fragments
11. Since love is eternal, death need not be viewed as fearful
12. We can always perceive others as either loving, or fearful and giving a call of help for love

Ho'oponopono

(ho-o-pono-pono)

Whenever a situation for healing presents itself in your life, consider invoking this ancient Hawaiian practice of reconciliation and forgiveness.

You simply say:

I love you
I'm sorry
Please forgive me
Thank you

You can state what needs forgiving (your perception of the situation), or you can simply say: *Please forgive me.*

This ritual can be used to heal relationships, health, money issues, legal situations, and more. What you are seeking is release rather than blame.

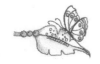

The greatest wisdom of all is inner wisdom.

Wisdom

I Create Adventure

I perceive, therefore I am

In my early twenties, I applied to be an air hostess with Qantas. I made it through several interviews, but in the end I didn't get a job. I was bitterly disappointed as that job was my passport to travelling the world and having adventures. It was only when I started taking long-haul flights as a passenger that I was able to thank Goddess for unanswered prayers. I would have hated the job, stuck in tiny aisles and being confined in an enclosed space with screaming babies and burping men. Not to mention having to look immaculate *all* the time. I'm a woman who is more comfortable working from home, writing books in her fleecy pyjamas than wearing stockings, high heels and hairspray. Having said that, I'm always open to a foreign holiday!

My eighteen-year-old daughter has just booked her first overseas adventure as an adult: to travel on her own to Estonia. What a joy to watch her literally fly into adult life! That sense of anticipation about adventure, possibilities, and learning more about the world is a classic archetypal energy of this house.

Astrologically, the ninth house explores themes to do with adventure, seeing the world, but also higher learning, such as philosophy. Here we consider what comes from experiencing foreign cultures and travel, but we're also likely to come across a love of higher learning, such as university life. This area also covers publishing and the sharing of wisdom far and wide.

In your own life, when considering how to create your day, give thought to where in your life you regularly have adventure. Perhaps it's on horseback or by reading travel magazines. Maybe you publish a blog to a worldwide audience, or maybe you study foreign cuisines to jazz up your nightly cooking. Mostly, ask yourself where you receive your wisdom and inspirational teachings from. How do they infuse your daily life? Indeed, are you allowing yourself to be nourished in this way? If not, why not?

This area of life is where we ask the big questions, such as "What the heck is this life all about?" It can be exciting to ask, but more often than not for many people the human experience can seem utterly pointless, infuriating, and like being on a meaningless treadmill.

What I have come to understand is that the meaning of life is….whatever meaning we give to it! There is no definitive answer, but I promise you that the more you live in the present moment, and treat each day as sacred, the less tormenting that question will be.

Symbols and Archetypes

As an astrologer, I work largely with symbols and archetypes, and use these to explore themes in my clients' charts. Of course, you don't need to be an astrologer to do that! In your daily life, take note of symbols that may appear. Learn to read the signs: butterfly, owl, rainbow, white feather, just to name a few. Seeing symbols and decoding their meanings is another way of knowing we're on track and living in alignment with our Higher Self. An owl, for example, signifies change. A rainbow is a gift from the Creator that good things are coming. What do you think it means if you end up at a crossroad?

Why not give your own meaning to symbols? For example, many people think that breaking a mirror is bad luck. If it happens to me I say "Wow, unexpected money is coming to me". I am *never* superstitious about walking under a ladder, and instead affirm: I am always lucky.

If I see a random butterfly (as opposed to hundreds gathering on my Buddleia bush), I consider it to mean that news is coming.

If you hear of whales or dolphins stranded on a beach, perhaps it is a message that you're out of sorts and away from your natural environment.

Maybe seeing an apple (aside from in your fruit bowl) is a message about fertility and abundance, while seeing or hearing a harp might remind you to get in touch with your spiritual nature. Seeing a sunflower might indicate wealth or ambition, while a tulip shows you the power of resurrecting.

In this area of life, we might explore personal growth, and work consciously to become the best version of who we are. Along the way, we may meet teachers who guide us and show us a new direction.

The greatest wisdom of all is inner wisdom. This call for adventure is the part of us that seeks meaning. It is both our eyes looking outwards, and our soul calling us to the inner terrain. We want to cross the horizon and discover new lands, either literally or metaphorically. And the truth is, it doesn't matter which one you pursue, only that you do.

As I was writing this chapter, I was thinking about my love of travel, and how very much I'd enjoy a holiday in the sunshine with my family. My daughters are adults now, and I'd really love for us to just have a week together free of work and other commitments. I had given no thought to how I was going to manifest it, but one thing I do know is that you don't always how to know the 'how or why' of things. I decided that I'd do a manifestation ritual as soon as I was sure where I wanted to travel to. The only thing I knew was that I wanted it to be somewhere hot, and in easy-flying distance.

Yesterday I won a family holiday for four, for a week, in sunny Portugal. It took about an hour or so for it to really sink in, but when it did, my levels of gratitude could be felt far and wide. What was really interesting is that yesterday morning I was walking through town and repeating the affirmation: *I am always in the right place at the right time.* Anyway, I stepped into a health chain store. I rarely go into this shop, preferring instead to support my local independent health store. However, I popped in there as my daughter had wanted me to scout some almond yoghurt. When I was at the counter, the assistant asked if I wanted to buy their magazine. Why not? I thought, and he added it to the collection of things I was purchasing.

I left town, pondering my affirmation, and was

surprised that I hadn't bumped into anyone I knew, which is most unusual on a Saturday morning. Later that day, snugged up on the sofa, I began to read the magazine. Something fell out of it: a scratch card. For years I'd heard my mother say she didn't like scratch cards, and she didn't want to 'scratch for her money!' I don't mind how the Universe wants to gift me so long as it doesn't involve pain or suffering or something illegal. I noticed the scratch-card prizes included an amount I was working on manifesting. I excitedly wondered if perhaps it was a winning ticket. It *was* a winning ticket, alright, but not for the cash prize. I won the overseas holiday! I can't say that I'm someone with a knack for winning prizes, but I do know this: when we're aligned to our higher vibration, manifestations appear in our lap easily and effortlessly. I was (am!) ready to enjoy some time in the sunshine with my loved ones.

Aromatherapy
Cedar and sweet orange

Flower Essences
Wild Oat, Zinnia, Borage and Shasta Daisy

Meditation or Visualisation Image
In your meditation or visualisation, imagine a ship sailing over the horizon. You don't know where it's going, just that it is set on an incredible adventure. Feel your mind open up to the amazing possibilities before you, all the while remembering the old proverb: one must have courage to lose sight of the shore in order to seek new horizons. Let your imagination take you to a new destination.

Healing Modalities

Bioenergetics, yoga, meditation, religious practice, self-reflection, drawing mandalas, Nature mandalas, create a treasure map (vision board), armchair travelling.

Affirmations

I am always in the right place at the right time.
I am easily able to attract the right teachers for me.
I experience love wherever I go.
God (Universe/Creator/Goddess) loves me.
This legal situation is resolving with ease and fairness.
I create the life I desire.
I understand man-made laws and universal laws.
My life has meaning.
I create my own good luck and fortune.
The Universe responds to my desires.
I learn languages with ease.
I have a wonderful vision for the world.
I love travelling.
I explore new horizons with excitement.

Heart Questions

Where would I love to travel to?
What is the meaning of life?
What is the meaning of my life?
Where does my greatest inspiration come from?
Who have been my greatest teachers on life's journey?
Have I been a teacher for others?
What is my philosophy of life?

Achievement

I Create A Legacy

I use, therefore I am

Before I'd even become a teenager, I had a deep calling to make a mark on the world. I figured that if I became a writer, I'd be able to weave my way in the world all the while staying at home with my children. Funny how life works out, because that's exactly what I've done, with various skips and dances along the way as I turned other hobbies and passions into careers. This part of the chart in astrology is what we know of as our social shorthand, career, or public face. It is where we leave a legacy, and are most visible. For many people, they don't have a career (and have no desire to have one). We all, however, have a part of us that is visible to people who don't know us intimately.

While the sixth house has to do with the details of day-to-day work (and the *invocation* of sacred ceremonies), the tenth is about the rewards and success that come with having a career, or a *vocation*. It is how we desire to be seen by others, as well as how we express our authority. It is our public reputation. Interestingly, we often look to the tenth house to get a sense of someone's relationship with their father (or mother, if she was the authoritative parent). Of all the things we manifest in life, this is where we are most visible to our community and world at large. This is where we discover our ambition. For many of us, though, we know this area of life more profoundly as our reputation. It is the world's opinion of us. How will you be remembered? How have you protected and provided for those in your world?

The Mountain Goat

In astrology, the tenth house is home of the zodiac sign, Capricorn. It is represented by the goat.

There are three types of goat: the *domestic* goat, which is happy tethered to a post and living with the comfort of familiar surroundings. There is the *mountain* goat, destined to get to the top. This is the archetypal 'ambitious' Capricorn who sees the goal and achieves it. The third type of goat, however, is the ideal expression of this energy. The *sea* goat takes the best of the material world (climbing to the top of the mountain) and combines it with the element of Neptune (ruler of the sea), which puts us in touch with the Divine. No matter how high a mountain we climb, if we're in touch with the Source then all our worldly achievements not only make sense, but give us a soul nourishment, too.

Aromatherapy

Bergamot, black pepper and lime

Flower Essences

Rock Water, Elm, Borage, Oak, Wild Oat, Scotch Broom, Sunflower, Blackberry, Gentian, Mustard, Mimulus, Larch, Aspen. *Wild Oat* is the essence of choice when you're looking for your true vocation or meaningful work. *Larch* is for resilience and confidence.

Affirmations

I have an excellent reputation.
I am respected for my quality and value of work.
Everything I touch is a success.
I attract wonderful opportunities wherever I go.
I attract my perfect clients/customers.
I am a winner.
There are plenty of customers for my services.
I establish a new awareness of success.
I love what I do.
I express my authentic self through my career.

Meditation or Visualisation Image

In your meditation or visualisation, seek out the highest mountain top. Step by step you make your way along the paths, sometimes defining your own path, and eventually you get to the top. There's no one else beside you. You've undertaken this journey on your own. Sure, there were companions to start with, and helpers along the way, but the closer you got to the peak, the fewer people kept you company. You have chosen this. When you arrive at the top, sit awhile and take in the view. Is this what you were expecting? Was it worth the discipline and determination of the journey? This roof of the world will project you higher than others, for all to see, but they won't see who you truly are. What did you bring to the mountain top? As the way got steeper and more arduous, what did you have to leave behind? You have reached the top, the climax. Is this what you wanted?

Healing Modalities
Adler (psychopathology), chiropractic, rolfing (structural integration), mountain climbing

Heart Questions
What is your legacy?
What will you be remembered for? Is this how you want to be remembered?
What will your eulogy say?
In what ways have you contributed to society?
Sum up your life in one sentence.
Write a list of ten successes you've had in this life.

Fellowship

I Create Community

I know, therefore I am

From the youngest age, many of my friendships have been with people who were unusual or who seemed unlikely companions. At five, my best friend wasn't someone from my age group but a neighbour in her fifties. At ten, I met a truckdriver named Bluey who read my palm, and we forged a friendship that spanned three countries and lasted until his dying day. He was in his fifties when we met.

This area of life is where we find our 'circle'. It's about friendship, and more widely it's about the love we receive from others (outside of marriage or similar intimate partnership). It is about our hopes, dreams and wishes, and knowing that these things can and do come true! It is also about our global community, and how we contribute to that.

When I read an astrology chart, I look to this house to understand not only someone's hopes and wishes, but also how they function in groups and within organisations. That is, how they interact with others in a group setting.

Do they belong? Do they find it hard to fit in? Can they speak up and have a voice in the world? When we connect with groups, our ability to attract opportunities increases.

Aromatherapy
Lime and blood orange

Flower Essences
Walnut, Star of Bethlehem, Water Violet, Chamomile, Dill, Red Clover, Scotch Broom, Quaking Grass.

Affirmations
I am lovable.
Love is everywhere.
I am open and receptive to love.
Others only reflect the good feelings I have about myself.
I love and approve of all that I am.
My dreams come true.
There is a group that is perfect for me.
I network easily.

Meditation or Visualisation Image
In your meditation or visualisation, imagine a circle of people in a Native American Indian tribe. They are all gathered around the fire. It's late at night, and they are joking and telling stories and playing handmade wooden flutes, and sharing what they've experienced during the day. Where is your place in this circle? Are

178

you actively taking part? How do you feel as 'one' within a group?

Healing Modalities
Group therapy, women's or men's circle, meridian therapies, acupuncture, astrology, energy medicine, radiesthesia (dowsing), homeopathy.

Heart Questions
How do I share my creativity with the world?
What groups do I belong to?
What is my role in a group setting?
In what ways am I actively reforming the world?

"We are what we repeatedly do."
~Aristotle

Spirituality

I Create Calm

I believe, therefore I am

Although many astrologers consider the 12th house to be the house of endings (and associate it with many negative things/places), as I understand and experience it, it's the house of completion. I also see it as our spiritual ancestry: karma…where we've come to make amends. This is probably my favourite part of the natal chart, for it is here that one can learn how to find sanctuary in spirituality.

I believe it is here where we find deep inner peace by focusing on the spiritual realm, and remembering where it is we all come from: The Source. We've travelled the zodiacal houses understanding our life's journey and human experiences, so it's only right that we have a place, an inner world, where we can understand that it's actually all an illusion.

What can cause difficulties in this area of life is our refusal to surrender to the Light within. Ours is a culture with 24/7 pollution: light, noise, activity. The twelfth house asks us to let go of all these, and to dwell within the silence. In many ways, to 'create your day', this is the first place you need to visit, not the last. If you consider silence to be your altar, then it is upon this pure vibration that you can begin to build the energy required for the other areas of your life.

Silence is our natural state. As Kahlil Gibran wrote:

You talk when you cease to be at peace with your thoughts. And when you can no longer dwell in the solitude of your heart you live in your lips, and sound is a diversion and a pastime. And in much of your talking, thinking is half murdered. For thought is a bird of space, that in a cage of words may indeed unfold its wings but cannot fly.

I consider this area of life to be the place of dreaming, for it is from here that we can create new beginnings in life. For some people, the twelfth house in astrology may be represented by places such as hospitals or other institutions which are considered to be behind closed doors. If we haven't nurtured our spiritual life, we may unconsciously end up creating visits to hospital to foster some much-needed seclusion.

By consciously creating the sanctuary you need for restoration and healing, the less likely you are to create 'space' through a hospital (or jail) stay.

Self-sabotage and unhealthy escapism, such as delusion, alcoholism and drug abuse, need not manifest in your life if you're regularly listening to your dreams, and honouring your intuition. At the highest level, the twelfth house is about feeling at one with the Universal energy. It is the search for divinity, unity and love.

Aromatherapy
White grapefruit and lemon

Flower Essences
Clematis, Rock Rose, Lavender, California Poppy, Pink Yarrow, Corn, Forget-me-not, Aspen, Lotus, Morning Glory

Affirmations
I allow the Divine to manifest in my daily life.
I am a mystic, and create heaven on Earth.
It is safe for me to incarnate in human form.
To a new baby: It is safe for you to be here on this Earth.
I listen to my dreams.
I am at one with the Universe. I have a right to be here.
Every hand that touches me in the hospital is a healing one.
Everyday I feel better.
I release the pattern in my consciousness that has created this condition.
I am healing perfectly.

We've travelled the zodiacal houses
understanding our life's journey
and human experiences,
so it's only right that we have a place,
an inner world,
where we can understand
that it's actually all an illusion.

Meditation or Visualisation Image

In your meditation or visualisation, imagine you're walking along a clifftop watching the sea. There is no one else around. You feel safe, content, and at peace. You enjoy the feel of grass beneath your feet, and savour the last few minutes of daylight. After the Sun dips below the horizon, you smile as the stars light up the dark sky. You are a child of the Universe. You feel connected to everyone, and everything.

Nearby, in the woods, a log cabin awaits you. Making your way there by starlight, you enter and then sit by the open fire, listening to the wood crackle and pop. By candlelight, you write down five things that you are grateful for this day. Nodding your head in appreciation, you acknowledge that all is well in your world. You feel connected to the heavens and Earth. You slide beneath the blankets of your big comfortable bed, sinking into bliss, and within moments your eyes are closed and you have drifted off into a peaceful sleep.

Healing Modalities

Keep a dream journal, meditation, intentional solitude, faith healing, A Course in Miracles, reflexology, devotional music, Reiki, spiritualist church, walking by the sea, past-life-regression therapy.

To see a world in a grain of sand
And heaven in a wildflower
Hold infinity in the palm of your hand
And eternity in an hour
~William Blake

> # If you don't remember your dreams, you are low in vitamin B6.
>
> Also, try spraying magnesium oil on the inside of your arms each night before sleep. You will soon be remembering vivid and colourful dreams.

Foods containing vitamin B6

bananas
watermelon
peanut butter
almonds
sweet potatoes
green peas
avocados
hemp seeds
spirulina
chia seeds
beans
chickpeas
prunes
wheat germ
sunflower seeds

pineapple
plantains
artichokes
water chesnuts
squash & pumpkins
Brussels sprouts
green beans
pistachios
figs
nutritional yeast
garlic
sage
peppers (capsicum)
kale
collards

Heart Questions

What is my soul's purpose?
Do I regularly connect with the Universe through Nature?
Do I listen to my dreams?
Have I ever experienced divine homesickness?
In what ways do I create sanctuary in my life?
When was the last time I actively sought solitude?
Have I experienced a stay in hospital? Did it allow me time to rest and be still?

Creating your day
when in difficult situations

There may be times when you or a loved one is ill, depressed, stressed, busy with little kids, and have no idea how to implement the ideas in this book.

If the only thing you do is start and end your day with 'thank you', that will be enough. Raise your arms up, open and wide to the Universe, in gratitude for all that you have, and all that you are. Do this twice a day.

Obviously, the more time and energy you can put into setting the tone for your day, with mindfulness, affirmations and conscious rituals, the more you will see the positive results around you.

No matter if you're a single mum with ten kids, or confined to a wheelchair, or a pensioner who feels lonely, you CAN create your day, and you have within you everything to make the world a beautiful, loving and generous place for you. If you've been able to read this book, and you can allow yourself to feel genuine gratitude for something or someone, then you're on the path to wonderful manifesting. Even if life feels challenging right now, there will be something in your memory (even if it was twenty years ago), that you can bring into your heart, and feel the wonderful energy relived. Use that energy to then manifest something else to be grateful for. Really visualise and feel the goal.

I would urge you to always be mindful of the words swirling about in your head, and the ones that come out of your mouth. Eliminate all forms of negative self-talk such as *I am broke*. Replace with:

I am open to…
I always have…
I have everything I need.

Seek out the positive.

When Family Members Don't Agree
There may well be family members who put a downer on every positive thought you have. Don't give up. At some point, the relationship will change. Stay true to your soul's purpose.

Illness/Diagnosis
Labelling an illness, disease or condition can be incredibly empowering for some people, and can give one a sense of finally being able to understand what is going on. However, a label can also inhibit, limit and condition us to be a certain way. I know from experience with certain health issues that discovering what was going on meant I could take necessary action for the right healing to begin. It was like stepping out of a maze of confusion and seeing things with clarity and understanding. I have also caught myself refraining from living fully because of such labels, and so have allowed myself the liberty of stepping away from constantly reaffirming that I have, for example, low thyroid, adrenal fatigue, high oestrogen, etc. Why? Because labels are only as good as our positive use of

them. As soon as they are used to limit us, we're asking for one thing: to perpetuate the story. We can't hope to change the script if we keep repeating the same thing over and over again.

Ask For Big Things

Don't be afraid to ask for big things in this life. I don't necessarily mean materially, unless that's what you want. What is your dream? What is your big, wild, this-is-my-life dream? Put it out to the Universe. Create your day. Create your life!

Increase your Life-Force Energy

The Greek word *thymos* means life energy. The thymus gland is known as the 'happiness point', and when working effectively can release negativity, as well as increase vitality, and bring about a sense of calm. It is part of the lymphatic immune system, and, particularly as we age, it needs to be stimulated.

A quick and simple technique to activate the thymus (and thereby improve happiness levels, raise your vibration, and strengthen your immune system) is to thump your thyroid. Quite simply, breathe in deeply (repeating a positive thought or affirmation, if you like) and with a closed fist gently thump your thymus gland. It is underneath the sternum (breast bone). Thump it for at least 20 seconds, and do this at least three times a day; more often if you're under extreme stress.

You will know when it's working because you'll become aware of a feeling of joy, and may experience a tingling sensation. This simple practice will stimulate the release of white blood cells by the thymus gland, which protect against contagious illness, disease and nurture the immune system.

Go Create!

Creating your day is so simple that it may seem impossible that these ideas can change your life.

You are only ever *one thought away* from creating your day, and manifesting the life of your dreams. Expand your field of influence, and radiate positivity wherever you go. Ramp up your fun, because the more fun, play and delight that fills your every waking day, the more pleasure you will experience.

It has been said that life is about using the whole box of crayons. Go on, then, go and draw your dreams in beautiful colours!

I wish you a life of joy, laughter, freedom, beauty, friendship, excellent health, meaning, adventure, creativity, abundance, the abiding love of a soulmate, a deeply profound self-love, and that you find gorgeousness in every single day.

Go in peace,
Veronika Sophia Robinson
Eden Valley, Cumbria, England
Full Moon in Virgo, February 2016

Have you received value from this book?

As an independent author, I would be most grateful if you could leave a review on Amazon or Goodreads, or perhaps send me an email so I can post your letter on my website?
Thank you so much. ~ Veronika

E: veronikarobinson@hotmail.com

About the Artist

Tracy Jane Roper

Tracy is passionate about art and its nourishment of the soul. Spending time in the woods with friends gives her the inspiration to create. She is deeply rooted in Cornwall and its changing seasons, and juggles being a mama to two boys with the occasional days to further her love of art. She also shares her passion with her children and her friends, and they regularly join in for messy fun. Tracy is a keen cook, forager, home educator, animal lover, pagan and Nature geek, drawing on all these influences to create in her everyday life. Find Tracy on Facebook at *WildLuna Art*.

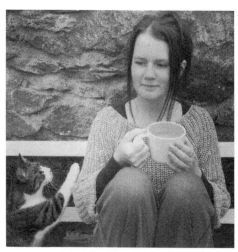

*Tracy Jane and her familiar, Connie,
enjoying time together by a Cornish stone wall.*

About the Author

Veronika Sophia Robinson

Veronika is the author of seventeen books (fiction and non-fiction), and has been a celebrant since 1995. She officiates blessingways, namings, weddings, funerals, memorials, and other rites of passage. A second-generation astrologer, she loves bringing the archetypes and symbols of this divine language into people's lives to be used in a practical, life-affirming way. Veronika has been studying metaphysics since childhood.

She takes pleasure from the simple things in life: leaves crunching under her feet, dewy cobwebs in the morning sunshine, rain falling on a tin roof, sunrise and sunset, moonlight keeping her awake, ripe mangoes, her husband's kisses (not to mention his perfect coffee), her children's laughter, time with friends, birds circling on high, intentional solitude, and cello music.

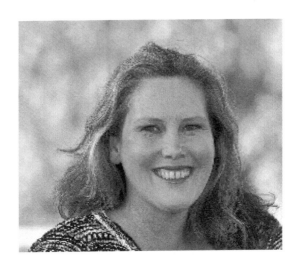

Other books by the same author

Fields of Lavender (poetry) 1991, out of print.

The Compassionate Years: history of the Royal New Zealand Society for the Protection of Animals. (RNZSPCA 1993)

The Drinks Are On Me: everything your mother never told you about breastfeeding (First edition published by Art of Change 2007) (Second edition by Starflower Press 2008)

Allattare Secondo Natura (Italian translation of The Drinks Are On Me 2009) published by Terra Nuova www.terranuovaedizioni.it

The Birthkeepers: reclaiming an ancient tradition (Starflower Press 2008)

Life Without School: the quiet revolution (Starflower Press 2010), co-authored by Paul, Bethany and Eliza Robinson

The Nurtured Family: ten threads of nurturing to weave through family life (Starflower Press 2011)

Natural Approaches to Healing Adrenal Fatigue (Starflower Press 2011)

Stretch Marks: selected articles from The Mother magazine 2002 – 2009, co-edited with Paul Robinson (Starflower Press)

The Mystic Cookfire: the sacred art of creating food for friends and family (more than 260 vegetarian recipes) (Starflower Press 2011)

The Blessingway: creating a beautiful Blessingway ceremony (Starflower Press 2012)

Baby Names Inspired by Mother Nature (Starflower Press 2012)

Cycle to the Moon: celebrating the menstrual trinity ~ menarche, menstruation, menopause (Starflower Press 2014)

Fiction

Mosaic (Starflower Press 2013)
Bluey's Cafe (Starflower Press 2013)
Blue Jeans (illustrated children's book) 2014 (out of print)
Sisters of the Silver Moon (2015)

Look out for these upcoming books:

Love From My Kitchen (gluten-free wholefood plant-based recipes)
Behind Closed Doors (second novel in The Gypsy Moon trilogy)
Apron Strings: reflections on being a stay-at-home mother
Babymoon: creating a sacred space after birth

Join the Community

Veronika invites you to join the I Create My Day
community on Facebook.
www.facebook.com/I-Create-My-Day

Share stories of the life you're creating.

I Create My Day notes

I Create My Day notes

I Create My Day notes

Printed in Great Britain
by Amazon

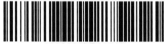

41323353R00115